Praise for *The Dental Diet*

"Dental health is almost a forgotten topic when we think about our overall health, but what if the health of our teeth and gums could alert us to problems like diabetes and Alzheimer's? Dr. Lin makes a powerful case for not only paying more attention to our dental health, but he makes the case that what is healthy for the mouth, is healthy for our whole being."

— **Robb Wolf,** *New York Times* and *Wall Street Journal* best-selling author of *The Paleo Solution and Wired to Eat*

"The future of medicine is interconnected in every way. The oral-systemic link is an obvious example of this greater trend, and I am thrilled to see dentists like Dr. Steven Lin leading the way in showing why we must work together to change the trajectory of healthcare worldwide."

— **James Maskell,** founder of Evolution of Medicine and author of *The Evolution of Medicine*

"*The Dental Diet* is an incredible resource. Grounded in new understandings of the critical importance of the oral microbiome to overall health, Dr. Lin leads the way with a unique action-based food plan that is a must-read for anyone wanting to enhance oral health and well-being."

— **Mark Burhenne, DDS,** author of *The 8-Hour Sleep Paradox*

"Dr. Lin is a complete breath of fresh air in the Lifestyle Medicine community. I've personally learned an enormous amount from his work, and I'm thrilled to see that he is creating a book to make this more available to the public. The dental-body connection is fascinating and completes a missing link for many people worldwide. *The Dental Diet* is a must for every patient and medical practitioner to read and understand for better overall health."

— **Rupy Aujla, M.D.,** author of *The Doctor's Kitchen*

"As an orthodontist that tries to help kids grow up with straight teeth, I know we have to go back to the basics: breathing, posture, sleep, and nutrition. From the moment of the first suckle, what we eat and how we eat it is critical to the final outcome of the face, airway, jaws, and teeth. Dr. Lin's prescription is just what the doctor should be ordering."

— **Barry Raphael, DMD,** founder of The Raphael Center for Integrative Orthodontics

"Crooked teeth are a sign of a deeper underlying problem. Dr. Lin's book provides a much needed look into the profound impact diet has on dental health. It also provides key strategies for parents to ensure their children have a diet that will support optimal dental and whole body health."

— **Dr. Michael Ruscio**, researcher, health enthusiast, and host of *Dr. Ruscio Radio*

"Dr. Lin's revolutionary leadership in nutrition and dentistry connected so many dots during our interview, we are thrilled his important better health recommendations are now widely accessible in *The Dental Diet!*"

— **Ashley Koff, R.D.**, and **Robyn O'Brien**, co-hosts of *Take Out with Ashley & Robyn*

"Dr. Lin's work is timely and addresses an important, upcoming field which few have ventured into thus far. Nutritional epigenetics captures the age-old saying of 'you are what you eat,' but he backs up this concept with up-to-date scientific evidence. I strongly recommend this book to students, doctors, dentists, and researchers in nutrition, dietetics, and obesity, as well as other healthcare professionals."

— **Professor Dave Singh, DDSC, Ph.D., DMD**, president of Vivos BioTechnologies, Inc.

"As an orthodontist, long ago, I saw the limitations of simply straightening teeth to improve a patient's smile. Over the last few decades, I have witnessed a paradigm shift in the focus of the dental industry through both speaking internationally and training thousands of dentists in the importance of functional airway dentistry. I believe the next step is for the profession to further integrate preventative steps, which is being led by Dr. Lin's nutrition program to address the malocclusion epidemic."

— **Dr. Derek Mahony**, specialist orthodontist at Full Face Orthodontics

THE
DENTAL
DIET

THE
DENTAL
DIET

The Surprising Link between Your Teeth,
Real Food, and Life-Changing Natural Health

DR. STEVEN LIN

HAY HOUSE, INC.
Carlsbad, California • New York City
London • Sydney • Johannesburg
Vancouver • New Delhi

Published and distributed in the United States by: Hay House, Inc.: www
.hayhouse.com® • *Published and distributed in Australia by:* Hay House
Australia Pty. Ltd.: www.hayhouse.com.au • *Published and distributed in the
United Kingdom by:* Hay House UK, Ltd.: www.hayhouse.co.uk • *Distributed in
Canada by:* Raincoast Books: www.raincoast.com • *Published in India by:* Hay
House Publishers India: www.hayhouse.co.in

Indexer: Jay Kreider
Cover design: Laywan Kwan • *Interior design:* Nick C. Welch • *Interior illustrations:*
Mesa Schumacher • *Interior photos:* © Price-Pottenger Nutrition Foundation, Inc.
All rights reserved. www.ppnf.org

Library of Congress Cataloging-in-Publication Data

Names: Lin, Steven, 1984- author.
Title: The dental diet : the surprising link between your teeth, real food,
    and life-changing natural health / Dr. Steven Lin.
Description: 1st edition. | Carlsbad, California : Hay House, Inc., 2018.
Identifiers: LCCN 2017029724 | ISBN 9781401953171 (hardback)
Subjects: LCSH: Nutrition and dental health. | Food habits. |
    Teeth—Diseases—Prevention. | Mouth—Diseases—Prevention. | BISAC:
    HEALTH & FITNESS / Diets. | HEALTH & FITNESS / Oral Health. | HEALTH &
    FITNESS / Healthy Living.
Classification: LCC RK281 .L56 2018 | DDC 617.6/01—dc23 LC record available at
https://lccn.loc.gov/2017029724

Hardcover ISBN: 978-1-4019-5317-1

10 9 8 7 6 5 4 3 2 1
1st edition, January 2018

Printed in the United States of America

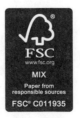

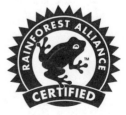

*To my family, friends, and countless inspiring
people who provided immeasurable love, support,
and guidance along the journey of writing this book.*

CONTENTS

FOREWORD

Throughout my career, in clinical practice, I've seen people deal with the consequences of lifestyle-driven diseases. For families, it can be tragic, because if the sickness has progressed too far, it's sometimes too late. Today the chronic disease epidemic is estimated to kill 40 million people globally. The U.S. healthcare system alone treats millions of people with type II diabetes and heart disease.

If we take a look at the mouth, half the population suffers from gum disease. And tooth decay is still the most common chronic disease in children. The health profession has long understood the links between gum disease, heart disease, and type II diabetes, including the fact that diseases that originate in the mouth have consequences for the entire body. Yet the health-care profession has failed to use this valuable piece of the puzzle to help shape our overall health.

Dental cavities can be a warning sign of how chronic diseases begin early in life. But more than being an indicator, oral health can be a means through which we *prevent* diseases before they cause long-term illness.

The conventional medicine model often treats oral disease and systemic disease separately with regard to the management of chronic illness, illogically fragmenting our approach to healing. Today functional medicine aims to understand the whole patient and not simply treat diseases from different organ systems in a compartmentalized way.

Dr. Steven Lin's program is instrumental in shifting our perspective to complete bodily health and getting to the root cause of disease. No longer will we see our teeth and oral health as merely comprising a warning system for issues with the rest of our body. Instead we will recognize that our teeth and oral health are functional and essential contributors to our overall wellness. *The Dental Diet* is the first and best guide to helping us understand the mechanisms of oral diseases such as tooth decay, gum disease, and crooked teeth and their effect on our general health.

One of the most instrumental shifts in modern healthcare has been recognizing the role of the gut microbiome in chronic disease. Food and nutrition all begin their journey through the body from the mouth, and Dr. Lin shows us how we can get in front of gut dysfunction by understanding the oral microbiome and the fascinating connection between microbes and the foods we eat.

The view that chronic diseases are mainly genetic is fast becoming disproven. *The Dental Diet* introduces us to the epigenetic model of crooked teeth, which illustrates that if we feed our kids the right food, the skeletal system will develop in the manner in which it was intended.

In my book *Eat Fat, Get Thin*, I explain how a low-fat diet is truly a mistake of the past, debunking the longstanding idea that low fat is heart healthy. However, this message still needs to break past our conventional healthcare system. Health practitioners must help guide people to reintroducing dietary fat into their lives. A vital approach of *The Dental Diet* is that it guides you through the benefits of dietary fat and fat-soluble vitamins.

A primary barrier for this progression has been our deeply ingrained mindset of thinking that fat is unhealthy. *The Dental Diet* simplifies the role of fat and is a groundbreaking step in preventing chronic disease by helping you to understand exactly which foods to put in your mouth.

I'm excited for this next frontier of functional medicine: one where doctors, dentists, and the entire health profession work in much closer collaboration, and one where we consider the whole person, utilizing lifestyle and nutritional changes as the true drivers of healing.

— **Mark Hyman, M.D.**, 10-time #1 *New York Times* best-selling author

INTRODUCTION

I'd like to tell you about the time I met Norman. He came into my dental practice in the south of Sydney one day with his wife, Mavery. It took only a few minutes with him to understand that Norman was a stoic but jovial man; he punctuated everything he said with a hardy joke or big grin. And that grin was something to see: he had only a couple of teeth left, so his smile consisted of gums and one tooth poking up almost diagonally across his mouth. Norman liked to joke that the one at the back was his eating tooth, and the one in the front was for the ladies.

But that day, there was a heaviness in the air that even Norman's larger-than-life personality couldn't lighten. Mavery wasn't laughing at any of his jokes, and she sat next to him with a noticeable look of concern. It turned out that Norman had been referred to me by his cardiologist; he needed dental clearance for quadruple bypass heart surgery.

Patients need dental clearance before major surgery for two main reasons. For one thing, bacterial infections in the mouth can spread to the rest of the body, so surgeons need to know that the person they operate on isn't more vulnerable to complications than they'd ordinarily be.

But there's another, more basic reason, and it's very telling. Pre-op patients also need dental clearance because if they develop a serious oral infection during recovery, the hospital will have a very hard time treating them. Hospitals, for the most part, don't deal with mouths and teeth.

The mouth is one of our most important organs, and its health is crucial to the rest of the body, yet most people don't appreciate this because medicine and dentistry have somehow become two separate worlds.

Norman's medical history was typical for someone at his weight. He was a type 2 diabetic with high blood pressure. When I examined him, I saw severe gum disease, which meant his last teeth would have to be extracted before he could be cleared for surgery. With the situation quite urgent, we were forced to take Norman's last teeth that week. We'd make his dentures while he was sent off to surgery, and we'd fit him with them once he was discharged from the hospital.

Norman's dental disease was severe, to be sure. But he wasn't as much of an outlier as you might think. I had been practicing dentistry for only about three years when I met him, but I had become used to seeing people with mouths that were much further gone than they should have been in a first-world, "advanced" society.

◆ ◆ ◆

Teeth have always fascinated me. I'm not sure what first drew me to them, but from an early age I was obsessed with keeping my own teeth squeaky clean. I was that anal-retentive kid who brushed on a military-like schedule, and I was upset by anyone who didn't share my enthusiasm. That anyone was usually my younger sister, Rachel, who was more of a daydreamer than a tooth-brusher.

We'd go into the bathroom at night to wash up, and I'd watch her just go through the motions. She basically sat there and sucked on the brush. I'd say, "You're not doing it right." I was all of five years old, and my mom still dressed me every morning, but I felt I was ready to be a tooth-brushing drill sergeant.

When we had our first checkup, my teeth earned an A+, and I left the dentist's chair very pleased with myself. When it was my sister's turn to go, she got into the chair very sheepishly. Of course I stuck around to observe.

When she opened her mouth, I saw a big brown spot on one of her teeth that I thought was a piece of chocolate. It turned out it was a huge hole.

I really gave it to her on the way home. My sister did a lot better after that, and to my knowledge she hasn't had a cavity since. But she, like most of the patients I see, needed that wake-up call.

As I grew up, I became more and more interested in health, specifically how nutrition affects the body and how it performs. I instinctively gravitated to a career in health care, and with my lifelong obsession with teeth, dentistry was a natural fit. I saw it as the perfect way to bring my love of health and nutrition together. I became a health practitioner to help people enhance their lives through their mouth. At least that's how I saw it.

In dental school at the University of Sydney, I learned skills that let us completely reconstruct people's mouths and teeth. I took it for granted that these procedures would improve not just people's mouths, but their lives, too. Then I started practicing, which was thrilling.

Every day I had new and exciting opportunities to apply my trade: crowns, bridges, veneers, dental restorations, dentures, implants, root canals, and oral surgery, including wisdom teeth removal. Each procedure was a triumph.

My favorite thing to do was to restore people's smiles. When we smile at each other, our bodies release endorphins that make us feel happy and warm; that small act is fundamental to how we communicate and live together. When a person has bad teeth and doesn't want to smile, it cuts them off not just from the very chemicals their own brain needs to feel well, but from other *people*. So for me, fixing someone's smile is like plugging in a Christmas tree. I get to see their confidence come back, right in front of my eyes. It's a powerful moment.

You spend your first few years as a dentist mastering these kinds of skills. Then, once you've learned how to do a procedure in an hour, you can start working on getting that time down so you can see *more* people in an hour.

But eventually, as you become more experienced at procedures, you begin to reach what we call the "clinical peak." You've maximized your efficiency with each patient and maximized the number of patients you can see in a day. Your hands can do no more. You're at capacity.

A few years into working as a general dental practitioner and honing my craft, I realized I was reaching my clinical peak. Every day I'd diagnose patients, give them treatment options, and then execute the treatment they chose. My work life began to feel repetitive. And since my work had become almost automated, my mind started wandering. But it always returned to the same subject.

At the same time that I was perfecting my surgical skills, I had been sharpening probably the *most* important skill a dentist can have: putting people at ease. Anxious, scared, or angry patients not only make our job harder, but are also less likely to take good care of their teeth on their own. As a dentist, you want to calm their nerves and boost their confidence in their ability to take care of themselves by getting to know them and relating to them.

But the more I got to know my patients, the more I discovered how little people understood dental disease and how it affects their lives. I saw plenty of patients who had fine educations and impressive careers but whose mouths were disaster zones. It was common for them to have broken, missing, or crooked teeth; swollen gums; and infected wisdom teeth.

I felt unsettled. I never expected to meet many patients who loved going to the dentist, but I was surprised by how many people avoided taking care of their mouths or simply had no interest in doing so. There were so many adults who felt as ambivalent about their oral health as my sister had when she was four.

It occurred to me that, in a way, they didn't actually have something to be interested *in*. Now more than ever, people generally know how to take care of their heart. They know how to take care of their skin and hair. They have some insight into how to protect most of their major organs. But they don't know how to take care of the organ they eat and talk with, the one that sits in the middle of their face.

Yes, they know that they should brush, floss, and avoid sugary foods and acidic beverages that can erode their teeth. They know it's smart to see a dentist at least twice a year for a checkup and cleaning. They know how to protect their teeth from damage from the outside. But they don't know how to make their teeth healthier from the inside.

So few people know how their jawbone grows, or why their teeth form the way they do. They don't understand that, just as you can eat certain foods to make your heart or your hair healthier, you can eat certain foods that will make your teeth and gums healthier. And they don't realize that there are a lot of things they can do to help set up their children's mouths for healthy growth and development. Nearly every child I saw in my practice had crooked dental arches, and almost half had some tooth decay. I almost never saw a teenager whose jaw had enough space to accommodate their wisdom teeth.

And I didn't exactly feel like I was part of the solution to any of this.

While I was diagnosing problems, I was never addressing the *why*. I diagnosed malocclusions (a misalignment of the teeth and dental arches), I worked with an orthodontist to straighten them out, and then the patient received a bill. But I could never tell them why their teeth grew crooked in the first place. I could never tell them why most of their oral issues had come about. I wasn't sure myself. Dental school had taught me how to *treat* these issues, not *prevent* them.

On top of it all, you need to be in the middle to high income range just to access serious dental care. Many of my patients need treatments that cost between $10,000 and $20,000, and it's not as unusual as you'd think for someone to need a procedure that costs as much as $60,000.

A diseased mouth can be a vicious self-fulfilling prophecy for lower-income people. They go for a job interview, and all people can see is their severely broken teeth. Their bad teeth stand in the way of their getting a job with a good salary—which, naturally, they need to fix their teeth. It becomes a vicious cycle. Without any way to fend off the initial onset of dental disease, they never stand a chance.

The same thought popped into my head with increasing frequency: *Am I going to do this the rest of my life?* I suspected that if I had to do root canals day after day for the next 30 to 40 years, it might drive me insane.

There was one dentist in the practice who was famous for throwing his instruments across the room if the nurse got him the wrong one. "Steven," he said to me one afternoon, "when are you going to buy me out so I can retire?" Compared with him, I was relatively happy in my work, but his words made me question the nature of my profession. How many extractions could I possibly perform in my entire life? How many cavities could I fill? And most important: *What real difference would it all make anyway?*

Over the past several decades, there have been phenomenal advances in dental treatment thanks to technology. Up until the mid-1900s, it still was common for a young woman to happily receive, as a wedding gift, money to have all her teeth removed and replaced with dentures to avoid a lifetime of expensive dental work.

Today we can reconstruct entire teeth with implants made from the same titanium that is used in spacecraft. And we use lasers and 3-D scanners to create tooth enamel so perfect that the naked eye would never tell it apart from the real thing. Soon we'll have advances we can't even dream up right now.

But we're still no closer to knowing why dental disease is so common in the first place. And that's disturbing. I spent my days chasing the problem from behind rather than getting in front of it and stopping it in its tracks.

◆ ◆ ◆

A few months after I met Norman, Mavery came to my office with the sad news that there had been complications during his heart surgery and he'd passed away.

Oral disease is both a warning and a cause of chronic diseases that harm the entire body. It saddens me to think that, by the time I met him, Norman's rotten gums and teeth had already led to a lifetime of disease that eventually left his wife a widow. His life was a painful testament to how our health care system and its attitude toward oral health have failed so many people.

Norman's death was a wake-up call. It made me realize that, as a dentist, I needed to widen my perspective of the mouth. How had we gotten to this point? When did it all go so wrong? While we were filling cavities and performing root canals, had my fellow dentists and I missed a sign that could have prevented Norman's disease?

I was determined to find the answers.

PART I

THE TRUTH IN YOUR TEETH

CHAPTER 1

WHY YOUR
MOUTH
MATTERS

Your mouth is the gateway to your entire body.

While we know how important our dental health is and undeniably love a great set of teeth, our mouths remain on the periphery of the modern conversation about health and well-being. When you look at the way we actually treat our teeth, it would appear that our oral health is unimportant to us, a fact barely hidden by the veneer of orthodontia and teeth whitening procedures.

Today, rotten teeth are so common that we consider them normal. According to the World Health Organization, tooth decay affects 60 to 90 percent of school-age children living in industrialized countries.[1] It is the most prevalent chronic disease in the United States, where 42 percent of children develop holes in their baby dentition.[2] In the United Kingdom, 26,000 children aged five to nine were admitted under general anesthetic for dental treatment from 2013 to 2014.[3]

Crooked teeth, also known as malocclusion, plagues our children. Approximately four million kids in the U.S. are wearing braces to straighten their teeth.[4] The total number of people with orthodontics doubled between 1982 and 2008 and rose by 24 percent in adults.[5] And if you are lucky enough make it to adolescence with an untouched mouth, your coming-of-age will likely involve some wisdom tooth pain. In the United States, 10 million wisdom teeth are extracted annually,[6] while the dental industry pulls in a colossal $129 billion a year.[7]

The numbers representing oral disease are simply staggering and reveal a modern health epidemic in our society that starts in childhood and spans our entire adult lives. The pervasiveness of dental disease has given us the idea that, as a part of growing up, we will *inevitably* experience decay, need braces, or have wisdom teeth removed.

Over the past few years it became wildly apparent to me that, as a dentist, I was focusing on the wrong thing. My training was based on fixing disease, not preventing it from happening. The flood of adults and children with diseased mouths continued to roll into my practice, day after day, with the same conditions. I felt as if my life's work wasn't significantly changing anything. Dental disease would continue to exist, no matter how many fillings I placed, no matter how many wisdom teeth I extracted.

We don't need another treatment that simply hides the problem; we need the solution. The uncomfortable truth is that all of these conditions occur simply because of poor diet. *The Dental Diet* brings this new paradigm to light and is the first book of its kind to teach people from all walks of life how to prevent dental disease by simply changing what they eat.

By following the dietary guidelines I've developed from studying human nutrition, epigenetics, and oral medicine, not only will you be relieving yourself from a lifetime of dental bills, but you'll be taking the best possible steps to improve your overall health and lower your risk of chronic illnesses like diabetes, heart disease, and irritable bowel syndrome.

Our focus on treatment has led to a poor understanding of how oral disease connects to the entire body and our health and wellness. In reality, what's good for the mouth is good for the rest of the body. The food program found in *The Dental Diet* helps to prevent disease not only in the mouth, but in your bones, gut, immune system, and brain as well. By following the recommendations found in these pages, you'll be setting yourself up for a lifetime of good health.

HOW FOOD SHAPES OUR FACE

Our modern experience with diseases like tooth decay and crooked teeth are placed into sharp perspective with a quick scan of the human fossil record. For anthropologists, jaws and teeth are like a time capsule taking us deep into human history. The dense lower jawbone and teeth are the sturdiest parts of our body, the parts most likely to survive undamaged in the fossil record. As a result, much of our knowledge of our ancestors is formed by posthumous dental checkups. Through the study of ancient mouths, scientists are able to re-create intricate details of our distant relatives, including their diet.

Fossil records tell us that dental disease was present yet rare among ancient Egyptians, and most of them had perfectly straight teeth.[8] Mesolithic hunter-gatherers had mouths with little to no cavities or gum disease.[9] More recently, anthropologists recorded indigenous Australians living in their hunter-gatherer state and observed their absence of dental disease.[10] The same has been observed in societies across the world, including native North Americans, South American Indians, and nomadic African tribes.[11]

Anthropologists have observed that the human jaw is a plastic structure that undergoes change in response to the demands of eating. However, it is alarming to see how quickly the modern deterioration of our jaw has spread across the human race.

Dental disease—as we know it today—appeared only after the Industrial Revolution, when processed foods became prevalent in modernized society. Our mouths were healthy for thousands and thousands of years, but this changed remarkably once the industrialized food system was introduced.

In nature, dental problems rarely occur. Our contemporary problems of rotten teeth and crooked dental arches are a sign of rapid and unnatural degeneration in our species that has appeared in the geological blink of an eye. It took only one generation after the introduction of the modern diet for tooth decay and crooked teeth to appear. As soon as we changed our food, our mouths also began to change.

WHAT OUR TEETH
ARE TRYING TO TELL US

There's an old saying that someone who has "their head on their shoulders" is generally intelligent, logical, and down-to-earth. The idea seems to have its roots in the simple observation that well-grounded minds require well-supported heads. Teeth are an excellent indicator of health—they tell us about the foundation of our skull, brain, and airway—which is why we humans are drawn to attractive teeth. A striking smile is usually accompanied by a classically square-like face with prominent cheekbones and jaw bones that can accommodate straight teeth, high-standing skulls, good airways, and upright skeletal posture.[12] It's these features that hopelessly draw us to the faces of famous actors.

Despite our undeniable obsession with good teeth, many of our mouths resemble a disaster zone. And when teeth are misshapen, other facial structures usually are, too. Crooked teeth indicate the poor growth of our upper and lower jaw bones, which not only house our teeth but also contain other crucial structures like airways, vessels, and the skeletal base for the brain. Looking at children today, you are likely to see long, skinny faces and slumped posture. Cramped upper teeth are a sign of a narrow palate encroaching on nasal airways, which can cause slouching and mouth breathing.

The mouth acts as the natural gateway to the body, a portal through which nutrition shapes our health. Up until recently, the mouth-body connection was vague and fragmented at best, but exciting new research has revealed the intimate relationship between the two. Over the past decade, our application of bacterial gene sequencing technology has found that the bacterial imbalances that begin in our mouth during tooth decay echo throughout our entire digestive system and body.

Our DNA, once thought to be the final word on our lives and health, is profoundly responsive to our environment. The emerging field of epigenetics shows how DNA molecules can be altered through the influence of the surrounding environment without changes to the code itself. The biggest factor is the food we eat. A soup of genetic complexity—based on the interplay of the epigenetic messages in our food, the genes of our microbial population, and our own genetic code—determines our health and longevity.

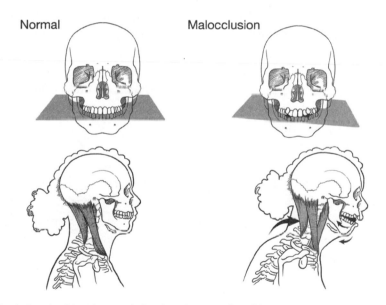

Normal Malocclusion

Fig. 1. Crooked teeth as a skeletal and postural problem

Dental disease is a painstakingly obvious message that something is very wrong in the body as a whole. Your mouth is your foundation for health, and the way you treat it is the exact way that your body will treat you back.

But with our distaste for dental checkups and our focus on treatment over prevention, we've failed to see how dental disease is an imminent warning sign of other health problems.

Society has trained itself to perceive the mouth as a remote part of health without any real influence on our well-being. Consequently, the medical and dental professions work as separate and disparate entities. Our health system is partitioned into silos, where dentists treat the mouth, gastroenterologists treat the stomach, neurologists treat the brain, and so on. As a society, we treat our bodies in the same manner.

We address chronic, lifestyle-related conditions that are on the rise, such as type 2 diabetes, obesity, and heart disease, with a self-propagating cycle of medication and surgery. General practitioners are trained to prescribe a pill for type 2 diabetes, so it's easy to lose sight of the fact that, like dental disease, it's caused by the modern diet. Nearly 10 percent of Americans, around 29 million people, have diabetes.[13] But while doctors and the pharmaceutical industry scramble to push out new treatments, processed food, which entered the food supply on a significant scale in 1965, now makes up 70 percent of the 600,000 food items in America.[14]

The most concerning thing is that these chronic illnesses are spreading to younger and younger age groups. We're plagued by digestive disorders (such as Crohn's disease and irritable bowel syndrome),[15] autoimmune conditions (like celiac disease, multiple sclerosis, and rheumatoid arthritis),[16] or other central nervous system problems (like autism, ADHD, and dementia)[17]—all of which, we are now learning, are significantly influenced by diet. Medicine's modern approach to each of these conditions is to diagnose and send to respective specialists who, in most cases, will prescribe a medication that only manages these symptoms and fails to treat the root cause.

In *The Dental Diet,* you'll learn how to harness the innate and powerful nutritional healing properties of natural foods. Instead of entering a cycle of sickness and symptom management, you'll learn simple methods for creating a tasty and nutrient-rich diet to ensure that you never need a dental filling or blood pressure pill ever again.

CHAPTER 2

THE MODERN DIET'S MISSING PIECES

THE CHARLES DARWIN OF NUTRITION

After years of clinical practice, honing my craft and approaching my clinical peak, I started to feel down. It seemed to me that my dental practice was all about treating disease rather than preventing it. How could I help people make their mouths and teeth strong and healthy, rather than just patch them up when something went wrong?

I went looking for answers in my textbooks, in the dental and medical journals, and anywhere else they might be. But there were none. I didn't feel like I was making a real difference, and I didn't see any way to change that. I felt a little helpless.

Eventually I felt so lost in my daily work that I decided to take a break from dentistry altogether. I traveled across Europe to ponder my future. What better way to rejuvenate than to surround myself with the beauty and energy of a European summer?

After trekking east across Europe, I found my way to the transcontinental Sarayburnu promontory and the bustling streets of Istanbul. The ancient Turkish port is a melting pot of religion, tradition, and modern Western influence.

One hot afternoon, after spending the day immersed in the rich culture of the old town of Sultanahmet, I returned to my hostel looking for a shady spot and a book to read. I went to the hostel's common room, which had a shared reading shelf where travelers left books they were done with and took books they wanted to read on the next leg of their trip. As I scanned the spines on the shelf, the initials *DDS* caught my eye. As in *Weston A. Price, DDS*. It's rare to come across a book about dentistry on *any* shelf, let alone one in a vacation setting. (I don't have the exact numbers, but I don't think most people pack dentistry books when they go on holiday. Not even dentists.)

Even though I was in Turkey to get away from dentistry, I couldn't resist pulling it off the shelf. The book was called *Nutrition and Physical Degeneration: A Comparison of Primitive and Modern Diets and Their Effects*.[1] It was a reprint of a book originally published in 1939. I had never heard of Price, but it turned out he was a dental professor, author, and clinician with a practice in Cleveland.

In the beginning, Price talked about his experiences as a dentist in the 1920s and '30s. He described how, over the years, more and more people with chronic disease came to his clinic and how they all seemed to suffer from oral disease, too. He sensed a relationship there.

Over a 10- to 15-year period, more and more of the children who came to him had deformed dental arches and tooth decay. And these children suffered from an alarming number of chronic diseases, like tuberculosis.

Price had a hunch that the rise in TB was somehow tied to the rise in oral disease. He suspected that there was a direct link between how bad a child's teeth were and how poor their overall health was.

From the very first lines of *Nutrition and Physical Degeneration*, I was transfixed. The words on the pages rang out with startling clarity, echoing my experiences with my own patients. Price framed dental disease in a way that, while not counterintuitive to me, lay outside the scope of my learning. More than 70 years before, he had shared my feeling that the conventional wisdom of medicine and dentistry was missing something—that reactive treatment was only one part of the puzzle, and that so many other questions needed to be answered. He wrote, "I am entirely serious when I suggest that it is a very myopic medical science which works backward from the morgue rather than forward from the cradle."[2]

Price had an uncanny ability to evaluate a person's overall health just by looking at their face and jaw. He didn't just see teeth when he looked into a mouth. He saw the structures forming the human face, airways, and digestive system.

His gut told him that teeth provided early warning signs of much larger problems. Through his research he discovered that the structure of the mouth was fundamental to the structure of the human body as a whole and that oral health was closely linked to overall wellness.

Price already had a theory as to the cause of the decline in overall health he was seeing. In his own lifetime, he had witnessed the technological advance of the way we consume food, which seemed to coincide with the rise in disease. Modern industrialization in North America, Europe, and Australia led to food processing that was widespread by the early 1900s. It seemed like a blessing for millions of people to have food that was much easier to obtain and prepare, but Price suspected we were paying a steep price for that convenience.

During the years he had devoted to treating dental diseases in his clinic, Price had also been working in his laboratory to measure the chemical components of different foods. His hypothesis was that processed, mass-produced foods were missing nutrients that were crucial for the health of the mouth:

> Modern commerce has deliberately robbed some of nature's foods of much of their body-building material while retaining the hunger-satisfying energy factors. For example, in the production of refined white flour, approximately eighty percent or four-fifths of the phosphorus and calcium content are usually removed, together with the vitamins and minerals provided in the embryo or germ.[3]

Price had heard that traditional cultures around the world were known to live in relatively good health, with fewer of the degenerative diseases he saw in the people of Cleveland. His intuition told him that these people, despite not having access to modern dental care, would have healthy teeth and mouths and that their diets would contain important nutrients that Western diets lacked.

It also told him that our forebears likely had well-developed mouths. He suspected that if he looked at the teeth and jaws of people historically removed from 20th-century America, he'd be able to link their poorly formed mouths and sickness to changes in the human diet.

With these theories in mind, Price decided to investigate first-hand the mouth-body connection in traditional societies and in the fossil records of the people that came long before all of us. He made it his mission to reveal that oral disease is largely dictated by the foods we eat, and that the state of our bodies is directly tied to the health of our mouths.

THE FACES OF THE EARTH

Looking to test theories that go against conventional medical and dental thought even today, Price devised a human research project of global proportions. Along with his wife, who was also his partner in research, Price would sail from Africa to the Arctic to see if traditional societies were actually healthier than modern ones—and if they were, what made them tick.

By traveling for the better part of the 1930s, just before World War II, Price was able to take advantage of perhaps the final period in history when people still lived in traditional societies all around the earth. His journey reached the heights of the Swiss Alps and the isolation of the islands of Scotland. He traveled across Africa; sailed to Australia, New Zealand, and the Polynesian islands; climbed the Peruvian Andes; and trekked through North America, Canada, and even the Arctic Circle.

While Price saw wide variations in the racial, cultural, and historical backgrounds of the people he met, one thing was astonishingly consistent: dental disease was virtually nonexistent. Dental arches were spectacularly well formed and teeth were more or less normal. His calculations showed that less than one percent of the people in these communities suffered from tooth decay, and he found crooked teeth to be equally rare.

Most surprisingly, none of these people had access to, or had ever even heard of, a toothbrush.

THE WISDOM OF NATIVE DIETS

In the early 1930s, Price and his wife landed in the remote Loetschental Valley of the Swiss Alps. It was home to people who until recently had lived in isolation from modern civilization and whose way of life was still rooted firmly in the past. Their diet revolved around the dairy products they could create thanks to the animals of the valley. And despite not having a doctor or dentist around, they were, for the most part, healthy and robust. They showed nearly no signs of dental disease, and skull records from the Valley showed few signs of it either. Price had a feeling that the dairy they ate held some secrets that modern nutrition had forgotten.

On every stop of his journey, Price gathered samples to measure the nutrient content of the local foods. Back in his lab, he discovered that the Loetschental Valley's cheese and butter, made from the milk of cows that feasted on the lush grasses of the Swiss Alps, showed remarkable levels of the fat-soluble vitamins A and D. It also contained a strange third vitamin whose identity would not be determined for decades. Price had a feeling that these were the crucial clues he was looking for.

In search of more evidence, Price visited a society that had been living in isolation since the Stone Age: the Inuit of the Arctic. Price marveled at their form and health, which stood in stark contrast with the people he treated back home. The Inuit exhibited practically no dental issues besides worn teeth from their tough diets. They had a distinctly brawny jaw structure. They lived primarily on animals they caught in the sea, and their jaws were so durable that many of them could carry enormous bags of fish clenched in their teeth alone.

Seal oil seemed particularly important; the Inuit liked to dip the fish they ate in it. In his lab, Price found that the oil was as rich in vitamin A as any food he had found.

Price began to see a pattern. The traditional Inuit and Swiss diets were based on direct acquisition and consumption of food. Price saw this as more proof that modern processed foods were missing crucial natural nutrients and making people very sick.

Price's research next took him to Africa. Despite the continent's reputation for deadly diseases, the people in the 30-plus tribes he visited there had strong, resilient bodies built for survival—and their teeth and dental arches were impeccable. He took particular interest in the Masai, a herder tribe he met in the Nile Valley. Just like the traditional cultures Price had visited in the Alps and in the Arctic, the Masai showed virtually no signs of dental decay and had fully developed, straight dental arches. They also showed no signs of heart disease, despite living on what Western society would consider a diet high in saturated fats.

Price was convinced that the Masai owed their health to their consumption of three fat-soluble vitamins that they consumed in the milk, meat, and blood they got from the cows they herded. The pattern he saw made him think these three vitamins not only played a key role in bone and dental health, but had a butterfly effect throughout the entire human body.

Price saw his suspicions about fat-soluble vitamins confirmed in the wild. He wrote of how African lions, in times of plenty, would hunt and kill zebras only to pick through the carcass to specifically eat the liver. The liver happens to be the body's largest supply of fat-soluble vitamins.

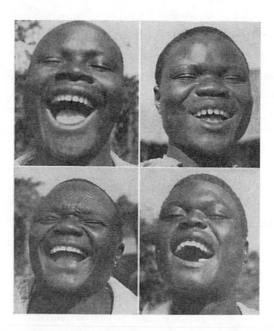

Fig. 2. Perfectly developed dental arches and facial features in African males[4]

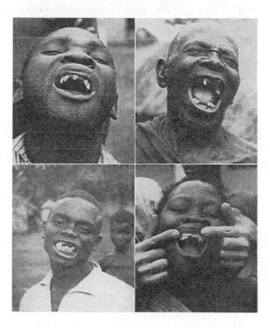

Fig. 3. Dental disease in African males who had access to modern Western food supplies[5]

The different clues Price picked up around the globe seemed to come together when he reached Australia. There he studied indigenous Australians, the oldest living human lineage in the world, dating back at least 50,000 years (as confirmed by genetic study in 2011).[6] In the indigenous populations he visited, Price again observed impressive dental arches and teeth without decay. The ancient records of their forebears showed patterns that were much the same.

But when he visited the colonies run by Europeans, Price saw a staggering rise in tooth decay and crooked teeth. And he observed that indigenous Australians who switched to modern foods rapidly developed modern diseases.

In the course of his world tour, Price met indigenous people in the Polynesian islands, New Zealand, North and South America, and the remote islands of Scotalnd. Each time he saw the same thing: people who lived in astonishingly good health even though they didn't have the luxuries of Western civilization.

After five years of traveling the globe, armed with thousands of photographs, food samples, and records, Price finally returned to Cleveland. There he would pull it all together so he could tell the world.

The missing pieces: fat-soluble vitamins

The one thing Price came back to again and again during his travels was that the healthy, traditional cultures he met all seemed to have diets rich in fat-soluble vitamins. Price was sure these vitamins were the essential ingredients that gave these people their outstanding teeth, jaws, and overall health. All of the societies he visited built customs into their eating habits that made sure they got healthy doses of these nutrients. His theory was that the fat-soluble vitamins served as "activators" that let the body utilize countless other important minerals and nutrients.

At every stop on his journey, Price collected food samples and preserved them so he could study them. The nutritional analyses of his samples revealed 10 times the number of fat-soluble vitamins found in contemporary Western foods and at least 4 times the calcium, in addition to other important minerals.

Price was able to identify some of the fat-soluble vitamins in the foods, but there appeared to be something else that led to the outstanding bone structure of the people he met on his journey. Price dubbed this mysterious vitamin "Activator X." The substance would be unknown for nearly 60 years, until it was discovered to be the fat-soluble vitamin K2. (We'll go into more detail on K2 in Chapter 4.)

A little-known fat-soluble vitamin that works in conjunction with vitamins D and A, K2 helps the body to place mineral into bones and teeth. It's crucial in the process of jaw growth and is fundamental to mineral balance in organs throughout the body.

After Price's death in 1948, *Nutrition and Physical Degeneration* fell out of print and was lost for the better part of 50 years. The book was far ahead of its time, but its reputation suffered because the scientific community couldn't see the validity of its claims.

There's no question that Price's methods were unorthodox and by no means perfect. Among other things, he did much of his research while he was on a worldwide voyage, and his samples and recordings had to be shipped thousands of miles. But just the same, Price had begun to chip away at something very important: the inescapable connection between the food we eat and its effects on our mouths and entire bodies.

As I flicked through the pages of *Nutrition and Physical Degeneration* on that hot day in Turkey, I began to look back on my entire dental career. My vision filled with crooked smiles and rotten teeth.

It would take many years to connect the dots, but I began to track what my patients ate. I found that most of those whose dental arches hadn't developed properly also had poor diets.

It all crystallized in my mind. For a long time, I had diagnosed and classified dental disease, but now it felt like I was finally getting to the root of it. It had been hiding in plain sight the whole time: *diet* was the biggest issue.

THE BEGINNING OF THE DENTAL DIET

Just as I had before I left for Europe, I saw lots of kids with mouths full of decay. I had to send many of them to the hospital to have their baby teeth extracted because they were so rotten.

To its credit, my dental training told me that these kids were consuming too much refined sugar and too many sugary drinks. But now it didn't seem to me that cutting down on sugar, by itself, could solve their dental problems. Price had theorized that the modern diet was missing nutrients that are fundamental to oral health; I suspected that, in addition to eliminating sugar, these kids had to *add* something to their diet as well.

Meanwhile, I was starting to have my own oral problems. I was suffering from unexplained and increasingly frequent bouts of tooth sensitivity. The pain was getting so intense that it became hard for me to eat hot or cold foods.

As the typical doctor hypochondriac, I bothered my colleagues for dental exams, after which they would always reassure me that there was no problem. Then I'd take the X-rays they had done on my mouth and scrutinize them myself. I looked for the slightest hint of any disease or abnormality, but I never found anything either.

At the same time, my body was sounding alarms. I had always been athletic, and I still worked out regularly, but now my weight was going up and down, and my joints ached more than usual. I was sick too often, and my skin didn't seem to heal as quickly. I chalked these issues up to aging, but another part of me said that they were coming on much too soon. I didn't realize until later that my body was in a state of inflammation.

Despite my nagging ailments, I thought I was pretty healthy overall, and even with some fluctuations, my weight was in the normal range. I stayed away from sugar during the day, and at night before bed, I liked to eat dark chocolate and low-fat yogurt with honey, which I had always considered a relatively natural, healthy combination. To the best of my knowledge, my diet was healthy, but when I looked closely at what I was eating, I realized that, like most people, I was eating foods that had far more sugar in them than I'd thought.

I was used to waking up in the middle of the night with a craving for something sweet. Now it dawned on me that I suffered from sugar addiction because many of the "healthy" foods I ate were full of sugar.

It was time to give my diet a complete makeover. The first step was to recognize which of the foods I ate were harmful and to eliminate them from my diet.

I read the labels on everything I ate. I gave myself a full sugar audit, counting every added gram. I also cut out bread and vegetable oils and stayed away from packaged foods. In short, I began to build the guidelines of what would eventually become the Dental Diet.

I did this for around three months. For the first couple of weeks, I could *feel* my body detoxing. The worst of it was about four to seven days in. I felt like a drug addict going through withdrawal; I got intense cravings and headaches, and a general feeling of hopelessness washed over me. But in a way, that was only fair. For years I had told patients who consumed more sugar than I did to "quit" it—without knowing how they should go about it or how it would make them feel. Now I was getting my just desserts.

The next step was to add foods to my diet that would give my mouth and body the nutrition they needed to perform at the highest level.

I began to research traditional diets, and the more I looked into them, the more I saw the wisdom in them. Traditional cultures had, over centuries if not millennia, structured their diets around the very foods that had the nutrients I was looking for. And that reminded me of my own childhood.

My Chinese grandmother had made a life in Australia by opening one of the first Chinese takeout restaurants in our town. Many of my earliest memories are of hanging around the restaurant while my dad helped my grandmother cook in the back; I loved talking to the steelworkers from the nearby plant who came in to get their lunch or dinner. There were countless days when I'd sit in the restaurant over a bowl of aromatic, steaming soup that had been cooked according to a time-honored Chinese recipe. Asian soups are usually made with meat that's still on the bone, and vegetables and organ meats are cooked with animal fats like duck and pig fat.

Even though my grandmother worked three jobs to support our family, she always was—and still is—as strong as an ox. I never saw her touch a sweet food in her life; she preferred plain hot tea when she needed something to make her feel good. My grandfather, ten years younger than she was, had a taste for junk food; he liked to sneak fast food and sugary sweets into his bedroom.

My grandmother said his diet would kill him, and unfortunately she was right. My grandfather went through a long period of chronic illnesses, type 2 diabetes, and kidney failure. Eventually he needed dialysis, and he lost the power to walk. What's more, his teeth were rotten and he barely had any left in the end. Meanwhile, my grandmother still has every single one of her teeth. "Of course I do," she'll proudly tell you while tapping them at the same time.

Thinking of my grandparents, I started to see the value of using animal fats in cooking or of adding an egg to basically every meal. And I began to appreciate the art of a slowly cooked and spiced stew.

My new diet

MEAL	BEFORE	AFTER (THE DENTAL DIET)
Breakfast	• Low-fat granola • Low-fat milk • Banana and dried fruit • Glass of orange juice	• 2 eggs spiced with turmeric, cooked in butter with diced tomatoes, red onions, and basil • Glass of kefir
Lunch	• Tuna salad sandwich	• Duck liver pate • Hard cheese platter • Avocado and spinach salad dressed with olive oil
Snack	• Fruit juice • Dried fruit • Muesli bar	• Coffee with full cream • Whole piece of fruit with nuts
Dinner	• Chicken breast • Steamed vegetables • Low-fat yogurt with chocolate and honey	• Beef stew cooked with marrow-filled bone, garlic, carrot, celery, bay leaves, and cilantro • Kombucha • Nuts and cinnamon in coconut oil
Midnight snack	• Packaged foods (like chips, chocolate, jams, and juices)	• None

Before I knew it, my health issues started taking care of themselves. My teeth felt stronger and less sensitive. My sleep improved, and my energy increased. I was no longer getting the common cold, and my sporting wounds healed quickly. The sugar cravings hit me less and less frequently, and I didn't wake up in the middle of the night anymore. In fact, I generally felt satisfied and never had hunger pains.

My taste buds changed, so I no longer craved sweets, and I again appreciated the full aromas of herbs, spices, and fats in foods. My hand–eye coordination at work was better. Even my brain seemed to feel more alive: my thoughts were clearer, and I was quicker on my feet.

My dental training had led me to doubt that my diet could profoundly affect my body and mind, but I was being proven wrong. So much was happening because I was eating better. I was a trained dentist, but I had come to this awakening almost accidentally.

◆ ◆ ◆

Right now you may be concerned that I'm going to tell you that, to stop dental decay, you need to eat whale's blubber or subsist primarily on cheese and butter. Don't worry—you don't, but it's important to understand why people ate those kinds of foods and how they contribute to good health.

The bottom line is that people used to shape their diet around the foods that gave their mouths and bodies the nutrients they needed to be at peak health. But now our diet is shaped more around convenience than around the foods we *need*, so we're missing those crucial nutrients. To gain back our health, we need to reshape our diets and relearn what makes food truly healthy—or not.

CHAPTER 3

THE ANCIENT WISDOM IN OUR TEETH

Imagine you go to your doctor for a checkup and everything looks good, but at the end of the exam she tells you that you need to have your pinkie toes surgically removed. It's not a serious issue, she says. Your feet simply haven't grown enough to fully support your pinkie toes, and they might end up causing you problems down the road. To make sure your feet stay healthy, your pinky toes will have to go.

Or imagine she tells you the same thing about your earlobes. Or your belly button. Or the tip of your nose.

It sounds absolutely ludicrous, right? It sounds like a science fiction horror story about the beginning of some horrible plague or the apocalypse itself. And yet, this is essentially what's going on with our wisdom teeth.

During the 20th century, wisdom teeth extraction became one of the most common surgical procedures in the Western world.[1] Today 10 million Americans have one or more impacted wisdom teeth removed every year.[2] And while there is some debate as to whether they actually *need* to be removed, there's no question that, generally speaking, our wisdom teeth don't seem to be growing in the way nature intended them to. But we don't give this a second thought.

According to Dr. Louis K. Rafetto, who led a task force on wisdom teeth for the American Association of Oral and Maxillofacial Surgeons, "Probably 75 to 80 percent of people do not meet the criteria of being able to successfully maintain their wisdom teeth."[3] Other experts have given lower estimates, but in the years that I've been practicing, I can probably count on one hand the kids who have developed fully erupted and functional wisdom teeth.

Accordingly, we now look at impacted wisdom teeth—and their removal—as a part of getting older. But when you think about it, it's actually very strange. There's no other part of our body that we so regularly remove.

Imagine that 10 million Americans really did have to have their defective pinkie toes—or earlobes—amputated every year. At some point we'd start asking ourselves if there was anything we could do to prevent our toes and ears from needing amputation in the first place. But when it comes to our wisdom teeth, we've simply never even *had* this conversation.

It's not like wisdom teeth removal is a simple procedure. Often the surgeon has to drill part of the jawbone away in order to expose a buried tooth, then saw the tooth in half before wrenching it from its bony catacomb. And when it's all over, the patient is often left with a severely swollen mouth and cheeks, and sometimes excruciatingly painful dry sockets. Anyone who's gone through this is probably nodding in agreement, and everyone else has likely had a relative or friend undergo the procedure.

You'd think that the difficulties of the operation and its side effects would get us to ask deeper questions about what's happening with our wisdom teeth. But on the contrary, we've spent very little time investigating *why* a person's wisdom teeth might end up buried in their jawbone.

And while it's true we can live basically healthy lives without our wisdom teeth themselves, those molars in the back of our mouth are a warning sign that something is going very wrong with our faces and bodies.

IT'S ALL ABOUT THE OXYGEN, THE NUMBER ONE NUTRIENT

Our epidemic of crooked and impacted wisdom teeth is a sign that, due to what we eat, our jaws are not developing properly. And *that's* a sign that the other parts of our skull, including our airways, aren't developing properly, compromising our ability to process oxygen.

Your body needs oxygen more than any other nutrient. This becomes very obvious any time you hold your breath for more than 30 seconds. Our cells need oxygen to be able to create energy. Everything our body does relies on oxygen.

When we don't get enough of it, it relates to all sorts of other problems—from snoring to ADHD to heart disease. The good news is that by changing our diet and practicing better ways of breathing, we can strengthen our jaws and airways. We can get more oxygen into our lungs and the rest of our body and start fulfilling our physical potential again.

But before we get into all that, let's look at how our skulls, jaws, and teeth developed in the first place.

HOW FOOD MADE OUR BRAINS BIGGER— AND JAWS SMALLER

Two to three million years ago, something started happening to our brains. Well, not *our* brains, exactly, but the brains of our very close, yet very distant, primate ancestors. Those brains started getting bigger and more complex.

We know that humanlike hominids eventually split off from our apelike ancestors and later evolved into us. We don't exactly know how this occurred, because we haven't discovered the so-called missing link—or, more realistically, missing *links*. But we do know that, in becoming "human," our brains exploded to become three times larger than chimp and ape brains. They grew from around 400 centimeters to 1,350 centimeters in volume.[4]

Larger brains gave our ancestors finer motor skills, which let them create and use tools; more complex language, which let them communicate and work together better; and the memory capacity and cognitive ability to learn from experience and modify their behavior so they could not just survive, but thrive. So they could become, in time, *us*.

Chimpanzee

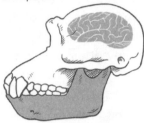

Early Homonin
(Paranthropus boisei)

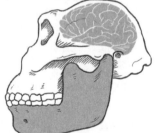

Homo sapiens

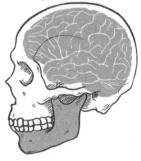

But these larger brains came at a price. Apes have large, powerful jaws, but as our ancestors' skulls expanded to accommodate their new brains, their jaws and teeth shrank. To this day, scientists aren't sure why this trade-off had to occur. Nor are they sure which came first, our smaller jaws or our larger brains. Perhaps they essentially evolved together. Perhaps it's an unanswerable question, like the chicken-or-the-egg conundrum.

One thing that's certain is that food was at the center of the transformation. Bigger brains need more nutrients to function. So one way or another, as the size of our brains and jaws shifted, our eating habits must have changed in a similarly significant way.

Fig. 4. The jaw-to-brain trade-off between primates and humans

Did cooking make us human?

In his book *Catching Fire: How Cooking Made Us Human*, British primatologist Richard Wrangham proposes one of the more compelling theories of how our brains, jaws, and teeth evolved: through our discovery of cooking. I had the pleasure of speaking to Professor Wrangham about his "aha" moment.

"One night I was sitting in my house, thinking of human evolution," Richard told me. "I happened to be sitting in the dark, in front of a fire, and I started thinking about how one of our ancestors must have been the first to have had that experience— sitting in front of a fire. All of a sudden it seemed obvious."

Wrangham began to piece together a theory that we had to become cooks before we could become human.

"We are the only animal adapted to eating cooked food. We are not as well equipped for eating raw food from the wild," he explained. "We have smaller teeth in relation to our body size than any other animal. And the same thing is true with our gut."

In their paper "The Expensive Tissue Hypothesis," anthropologists Leslie C. Aiello and Peter Wheeler argue that a smaller gut was key to our evolution because it lets the body spend less energy processing food and more energy fueling the brain. They say that a whopping 25 percent of our energy goes to our massive brain.[5] "It needs to come from somewhere," Wrangham said.

For the most part, that somewhere is the gut. Under Wrangham's theory, when we discovered cooking, it was as if we began to make a surrogate set of teeth and gut for ourselves. Cooking does a lot of the work that larger teeth and a larger gut would do; it makes food easier to break down, digest, and get nutrients from. (For example, cooked eggs are more than 90 percent digestible, while raw eggs are only 50 to 60 percent digestible.) As a result, our jaws, teeth, and gut shrank, freeing up more resources for our nutrient-greedy brains.

"The difference between a chimp and us is that our gut is small and our brains are big," Wrangham told me. "Across primates, smaller guts are associated with larger brains. The question then is, how long has the gut been this small?"

From rib and pelvis fossils, we know that we have the same size gut as *Homo erectus*, who evolved from *Homo habilis* around 1.8 million years ago. *H. erectus* was the first hominid to appear more human than apelike and had small teeth like us, too. "So," Wrangham said, "it seems like a no-brainer that we must have been cooking all that time."

We chew food with our jaws and teeth to change its shape and make it easier to digest. Under Wrangham's theory, food itself changed the shape of our jaws and teeth.

Wrangham's theory fits in with two key shifts in our physiological history. The first shift took place when we started moving away from a mainly vegetarian diet and started eating meat. The second was when we began to further feed our hungry brains by cooking our food.

Cooking is sort of like a surrogate digestive system; it breaks down the chemical structure of food and makes its nutrients more available to the body. Our ancestors' new, lower-energy digestive systems and smaller jaws let their bodies devote more resources to their brains, which grew bigger.

At the same time we decreased the physical work required of our jaws and teeth. Apes spend up to 17 hours a day using their huge jaws to chew on raw branches, leaves, and twigs. Once our ancestors started eating cooked meat and pounding and cutting their food with tools, they were in less need of the large teeth and heavy jaw muscles needed to grind nutrients out of plants. And once they started cooking their food, their digestive system didn't need to take up as much of their body's energy.

Maybe we'll never know *exactly* how it all happened. (It's ironic that, of all of our body parts, our *mouth* keeps such a secret.) What is certain is that diet played an important role in how we became human.

Unfortunately, it also played a starring role in our crooked teeth. . . .

Where it all went wrong:
Crooked teeth are a strictly modern problem

It's been suggested that impacted wisdom teeth might somehow be a side effect of our jaws shrinking to make room for bigger brains, that wisdom teeth were basically squeezed out of ancestors' jaws—and continue to be squeezed out of ours—to make way for even more neurons. In other words, that they're collateral damage of our own evolution.

But the fossil record doesn't bear this out.

Archaeological skull records indicate three points in human history where we can measure changes in our jaws and teeth:

1. Around two million years ago, when we separated from primates, our jaws shrank to modern human sizes.

2. Approximately 10,000 to 14,000 years ago, during the agricultural revolution, we began suffering from modern tooth decay.

3. Around 200 to 300 years ago, during the Industrial Revolution, we began suffering from malocclusion and wisdom teeth impaction.

Weston Price described just how sudden these changes were. "It is a matter of concern," he wrote, that if a scale were extended a mile long and the decades represented by inches, there would apparently be more degeneration in the last few inches than in the preceding mile."[6]

We had our big, new brains long before we had wisdom teeth problems. So it doesn't seem as if we needed to squeeze them out to gain an evolutionary advantage. Wisdom teeth stopped fitting into our jaw during the Industrial Revolution— after we started eating mass-produced, processed foods. Since then we've ground, refined, bleached, and packaged our food to the point where it would be nearly unrecognizable to our hunter-gatherer relatives. Since then, our wisdom teeth problems have only gotten worse.

Anthropologist Robert Corruccini has looked at thousands of modern and ancient human jaws and teeth. He's also studied contemporary urban and rural populations in Kentucky and found that dental crowding was linked to the adoption of a modern diet over a traditional one.[7] Corruccini attributes malocclusion directly to the consumption of soft, processed foods, which are much more prevalent in modern diets. He calls malocclusion the "malady of civilization."[8]

If our modern diet brought us only impacted wisdom teeth and malocclusion, that would be bad enough. But it also changes our skeletal posture, breathing, ability to metabolize oxygen—and even the very shape of our face.

THE BONY ARCHITECTURE OF EXPRESSION

No matter how it came to evolve, the underlying architecture of our faces adheres to a very specific and strict formula, even while our bodies come in a virtually unlimited number of shapes and sizes. To give us the ability to breathe, chew, swallow, speak, smile, and do everything else we do with our faces and heads, our skulls are designed in a very specific way.

The human skull consists of the brain casing and facial bones, 22 bones altogether.[9] Two of these bones are arguably more important than the rest, since they are most responsible for the form of the face, the ability to chew, and the structure of the airways. These bones are the maxilla, the upper jawbone, and the mandible, the lower jawbone.

Many people think that the jaw is simply a mechanical device that allows us to crush and chew food, but the truth is that it does so much more. In one way or other, the jaw has a significant effect on every other organ in the body.

THE MAXILLA

The maxilla, or upper jaw, forms the middle of the face. Its outer surface shapes the cheekbones, and its inner cavity houses the maxillary sinus. Its upper surface forms the walls and floor of the nasal cavity and the floor of the eye sockets. Its lower border holds the upper teeth and also forms the palate of the mouth. As the center of the face, the maxilla is crucial to eating and breathing.

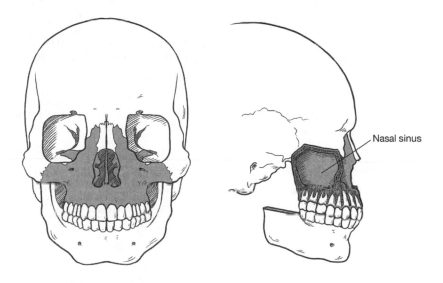

Fig. 5. The maxilla (upper jaw) bone

When the maxilla doesn't develop properly

If the maxilla fails to expand properly in one of the three dimensions of growth (height, width, depth), it can lead to problems including obstructed airways and crooked dental arches. And, as you might have guessed by now, it can also lead to impacted wisdom teeth.

At around 12 years of age, the upper wisdom teeth develop in the upper back portion of the maxilla. As part of this process, the maxillary sinus remodels itself by converting part of its hollow border into the bone that will house the upper wisdom teeth. When the remodeling doesn't occur properly, there's not enough space for the wisdom teeth to erupt; this is why, as discussed above, so many people end up needing wisdom tooth extraction surgery. And in some people, the wisdom teeth never form at all.

Wisdom tooth extraction is often necessary because impacted wisdom teeth can potentially lead to very severe issues. For instance, they can press up in awkward angles against the teeth in front of them, which can cause decay on the tooth in front, potentially leading to loss of both the wisdom tooth and the second molar. They can also develop while buried in the bone and can be even entwined with the nerve that runs through the jawbone (the inferior alveolar nerve). This is a nightmare for oral surgeons who have to try and retrieve them without damaging the nerve and causing permanent numbness in the lip or tongue.

Improper development of the maxilla and the mandible (lower jawbone) also leads to crooked teeth. Simply put, the jaw bones are like platforms that the teeth have to grow out of; when the platforms aren't the right size or they're misshaped in some way, the teeth can't grow in straight. It's as if the maxilla and mandible are the concrete foundations of seating sections in a stadium. If the concrete is warped or distorted or the foundation is just too small, you can't install the seats in neatly aligned rows. They end up bunching together or jutting out at odd angles.

Since the bones in the skull are so intimately connected with one another, a misshapen maxilla can lead to issues in other areas of the face and skull, such as the eye sockets and nasal sinuses. If the maxilla is irregular, the entire floor of the eye sockets may be underdeveloped, distorting the eyeball and leading to eyesight issues like astigmatism or myopia.

How a misshapen maxilla can put you on an (unintentional) oxygen diet

One of the most important principles of the Dental Diet is that oxygen is the number one nutrient. As humans, we're designed to gather oxygen primarily by breathing through our nose.

A normal nasal passage is designed to slow down airflow in the sinuses; to warm and humidify the air; and to allow it to mix with nitric oxide (NO), which increases oxygen intake in the lungs.[10] When people breathe through the mouth, their lungs get dry, unfiltered air and no nitric oxide. That means their body is constantly starved of oxygen, the lack of which can damage their heart muscles, brain tissue, and potentially every cell in their body.

An improperly formed maxilla may also have a deviated septum and narrow, obstructed nasal passages, airways that are essential to our breathing. When people have a high palate with crooked upper teeth, their ability to breathe through their nose can be compromised.

Usually when we talk about diet and nutrition, we're talking about food. But oxygen is easily the most important nutrient we consume. Our bodies need it literally every second of every day, our entire life.

One way to help to get the right amount of oxygen, is to make sure your mouth, tongue, and airways are strengthened and toned. Among other things, that means giving your mouth, tongue, and jaws the right exercise. We'll look later at exercises to help you breathe nasally. One of the simplest is to eat whole, fibrous, and even tough foods.

THE MANDIBLE

Commonly referred to as "the jawbone," the mandible is the largest and strongest bone in the face. It houses the lower teeth and connects to the base of the skull to form two sliding hinge joints, called the temporomandibular joint (TMJ), which opens and closes the mouth. The mandible also provides the base for the muscles that support and control the tongue and throat, and in turn swallowing and breathing.

Like the maxilla, the mandible undergoes a complex remodeling process as it grows in width, length, and height. During adolescence, the mandible needs to add at least 35 millimeters of bone behind the second molar to make room for the lower wisdom teeth.[11] If it doesn't, the wisdom teeth won't be able to erupt.

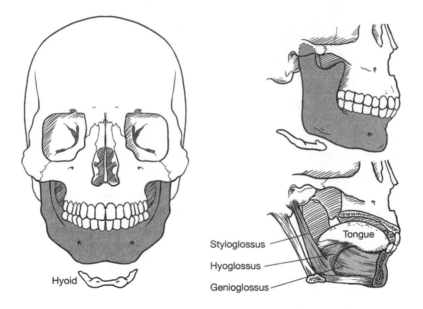

Fig. 6. The mandible (lower jaw) bone

How the mandible can cause sleep apnea and other breathing problems

Just like the maxilla, the mandible influences a lot more than teeth. While the maxilla bone forms the nasal passages, the mandible (lower jawbone) shapes the lower airways, including the soft palate (the back of the throat). Probably most crucially, the tongue sits inside of it like a hammock.

The tongue is made up of a complex group of muscles that connect to the mandible, the soft palate, and a horseshoe-shaped bone at the front of the neck called the hyoid bone. These muscles act as a support structure for the airway. At rest, the tongue should sit on the roof of the mouth, causing the airway to be tense and strengthened, holding it open. But when the palate is narrow and the tongue sits at the bottom of the mouth, the muscles don't hold the airway open the way they should.

There's also less space for the tongue when the mandible can't properly house the wisdom teeth. This can lead to poor tongue posture, where the tongue falls back into the throat instead of staying against the roof of the mouth, which can reduce muscle tone. A tongue with a lack of muscle tone can block the airway and hamper breathing, starving the lungs of important oxygen.[12] This condition can worsen during sleep, leading to issues like sleep apnea (pauses in breathing during sleep).[13]

The biology—and math—behind the human face

In the opening of Dan Brown's best-selling novel *The Da Vinci Code*, a young cryptologist discovers that before her grandfather died from stab wounds, he scribbled a series of numbers on the ground: 1, 1, 2, 3, 5, 8, 13, 21. It turns out that this is the Fibonacci sequence, a series where the ratio of two numbers are the same as the ratio of their sum to the larger two quantities. When you divide the ratio of any number above two in the sequence by the sum of the larger of the two quantities, you get 1.62, also known as the Greek letter phi (φ). Phi represents the "golden ratio," which has been found to govern the biological growth of organisms in nature.

The petals, branches, and roots of many plants, for instance, grow in a mathematical pattern based on the golden ratio, which maximizes sunlight and energy exposure (yet another possible example of why beauty is often associated with health). This pattern is said to be used in architectural wonders like the Parthenon in Athens and Notre Dame Cathedral in Paris. Even Beethoven's Fifth Symphony uses the principles of the golden ratio.

And according to one doctor, the shape of our faces is based on the golden ratio as well. Dr. Stephen Marquardt, former Chief of facial imaging at UCLA, has calculated a matrix that serves as a guide to what we regard as "healthy proportions" in the human face. While the applications of the formula for human beauty are controversial, the principles of facial development seem to abide by these laws of nature. Studies have shown that humans have a built-in affinity for certain faces. Babies, for example, gaze longer at "more attractive" faces compared to others, and may recognize them faster.[14]

The science and mathematics of facial beauty still remain a mystery. However, it's clear that the shape of the jaw dictates the proportions of the face and indicates well-developed airways and a healthy supply of oxygen to the brain. We may have an inner program that directs us to find people with well-proportioned faces attractive, or instinctively view them as healthier and more fit for reproduction.

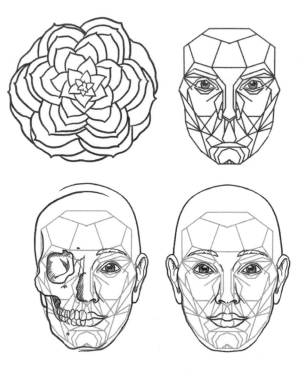

Fig. 7. Marquardt's Mask and the mathematical proportions of facial beauty

HOW OUR DIET CAN HURT OUR JAW AND FACIAL GROWTH

Our modern diet doesn't lead just to malocclusion. It also hampers our jaw and facial muscles and, in turn, our breathing.

Weightlifters go to the gym to lift heavy weights because they know that will cause their joints and muscles to grow strong. Our jaw joint is no different. Just like any other joint in our body, it needs stimulation to grow in the right way.

Most of our craniofacial growth is done by the age of 12. But the jaw continues to grow and develop in significant ways until 18, and continues to develop and change in smaller ways throughout our lifetime.

One aspect of bone growth is called appositional growth, where the bone grows in thickness. If there's one observation I've made during my years as a dentist, it's that people who grew up on farms or on traditional diets tend to have thicker and more robust jawbones.

The best example is a baby who is breastfed as opposed to bottle-fed. A newborn that latches on to a mother's breast is naturally induced to use its tongue muscles to push the nipple to the roof of its mouth. Because the roof of the mouth is soft like wax, this action will flatten and broaden the palate, making space for the upper teeth. Children who don't breastfeed are more likely to have a high palate and crooked teeth.[15]

Studies show that when we eat a more refined, processed diet, our palates don't seem to develop as well as those of our hunter-gatherer ancestors, who ate a more natural diet full of roughage.[16]

The health of our jaw, facial structure, and airways starts with what we eat.

HOW OUR TEETH
ARE LINKED TO BREATHING

Orthodontia in the 20th century was all about giving kids a straight smile by aligning the "social six," the six front teeth on the upper and lower jaw. The standard practice was to wait until children were 12 or 13 years old—after their jaw had finished growing—extract their premolar teeth, and fit them with braces that would straighten their crowded dental arches. Today this practice is still quite prevalent.

But in recent years, we've learned that the growth of the jaw is not some random roll of the dice. The shape of our face is tightly connected to the development of the muscles that let us breathe, chew, and swallow. Waiting until the jaw is finished developing to straighten the teeth with braces wastes valuable time that could be spent helping the jaw develop properly in more natural ways.

For that to happen, the child's tongue must sit at the top of the mouth, against the palate, which puts pressure on the palate to expand and grow.[17] The child must also breathe through the nose. The flow of air through the nasal passage stimulates the maxilla to keep growing outward and helps to lower and broaden the palate.[18]

While research outlining these links dates back to the 1970s,[19] the notion that breathing plays a role in crooked teeth has generally not been applied in the practice of orthodontia. In fact, there's a new school of thought that extraction orthodontia may compound these problems by compromising breathing even more. If a patient has had teeth extracted to straighten the dental arch, a contracted maxilla can lead to jaw joint problems, sleep-disordered breathing, and a host of other issues, all in the name of a straight smile, or bite.

The muscles of jaw expansion and breathing

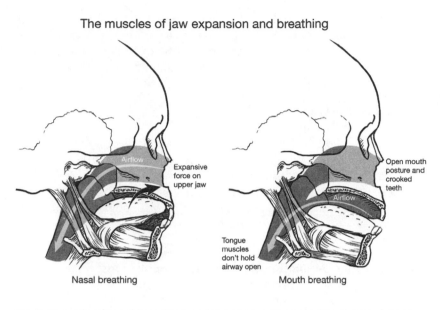

Fig. 8. The role of nasal breathing and the tongue in expanding the jaw bones

How to keep your face and jaw healthy

It's estimated you will take upwards of 20,000 breaths per day. That's a staggering number. Then there are the dozens if not hundreds of bites you take every day. Needless to say, breathing and chewing are very influential on the growth of your jaw and teeth. It's as if they're caught in a never-ending soccer match, constantly being kicked about by the forces of your breathing, tongue posture, and mouth muscles.

To help your jaw and teeth develop properly, you need to get those forces in line. Let's look at some quick and easy breathing and chewing exercises that will help you do that.

Breathe through your nose, not your mouth
Before we even consider vitamins and minerals, it's easy to forget that the most important nutrient for our body is oxygen. As humans, with large, oxygen-hungry brains, we're designed to breathe through the nose. Perhaps the best proof of this is found in children. When babies breastfeed, they're conditioned to breathe through the nose. This transfers the flow

of air from the mouth to the nasal sinuses and helps widen the babies' upper jawbone and palate to properly house their upper teeth. When children are taught to breathe through their nose, their jaws develop as they should and, as a result, their teeth grow in straighter.

Speak, chew, and swallow correctly
Breathing routines, vocal exercises, and tongue exercises will help you change the habits of the muscles in your face and jaw joints. When these muscles function properly, you'll also instinctively train yourself to breathe and swallow correctly. This helps to make sure you breathe properly during sleep and, in turn, this takes pressure off your spine and neck, improving your posture and preventing long-term neck and back problems.

Keep your jaw joints healthy with raw, tough foods
After you start breathing and swallowing correctly, you can start exercising your jaw to develop the muscles of mastication (chewing) that strengthen your jawbone and provide the architecture for your airways. Since you can't take your jaw to the gym, the best way to strengthen it is to eat raw, tough foods like carrots and celery with every meal. They'll keep your jaw joints strong and healthy.

A FUNCTIONAL APPROACH TO THE HEALTH OF OUR TEETH AND AIRWAYS

Today we are fortunate that dentistry can intervene in our skeletal growth, reducing the need for tooth extraction. Expansive, airway-focused orthodontics can steer jaw growth to help properly develop the face and airways. This type of orthodontics doesn't just give people straight teeth; it gives them the ability to breathe correctly.

Lactation consultants, myofunctional therapists, airway orthodontists, sleep physicians, and ENTs are all part of this multidisciplinary approach to facial growth. It lets us shape children's dental and facial development from a much earlier age and intervene more effectively when the growth of the skull is stunted.

Dr. Derek Mahony, a friend and colleague, is a Sydney-based orthodontist who recalls how he became convinced that crooked teeth didn't need to be extracted before they could be fitted with braces. After training to be a dentist at the University of Sydney, Dr. Mahony moved to London, where he practiced at the National Health Service (NHS). There he worked with a dentist who practiced early intervention orthodontics, and it inspired him. He decided to attain a specialty in orthodontics at the Eastman Dental Hospital. But the training was almost completely focused on extraction orthodontics—pulling out teeth to create the perfectly straight "bite."

When he returned to Sydney, Dr. Mahony was introduced to the work of facial orthodontic pioneers like Drs. John Mew and Skip Truitt. They taught him about the craniofacial growth approach to orthodontics. In this approach, the facial bones are expanded with the view that teeth grow with the entire facial complex. That's opposed to reactionary orthodontics, which in extreme cases takes four premolar teeth out and pulls the maxilla back, contracting its size and thus compromising the airways.

Further studies are needed to confirm this relationship between breathing disorders and extraction orthodontics.[20] But studies of identical twins who have had extraction and craniofacial orthodontics, respectively, show that those who undergo the craniofacial method have more well-developed facial structures than their conventionally treated siblings.[21]

Now, after 25 years of practice, training dentists and lecturing to the dental community worldwide, Dr. Mahony is part of a new age of dental treatment built around the idea that once you correct breathing, tongue posture, and facial muscle habits, the face and teeth grow as they should.

When we treat crooked teeth, or teeth that don't have room to grow, as a purely cosmetic issue, potentially much more serious health issues slip under our radar. I see the consequences of this in my dental practice daily—not only in older people like Norman, but also in younger patients whose breathing issues and other health problems are, sadly, only beginning.

THE BREATHING EPIDEMIC

Sleep is your body's chance to shut down various processes that have been working hard throughout the day so they can rest and recharge. Most important, it's your brain's time to rejuvenate itself. During sleep, your brain undertakes a "self-cleaning," removing metabolites and cellular toxins that have built up throughout the day.

Your body tightly protects your brain cells from outside threats by walling them off with the blood-brain barrier, which separates the blood that circulates in your body from the fluids in your brain and spinal cord tissue. It's the brain's filter for harmful substances. Research has found that another barrier exists inside the brain's cells. Normally cerebrospinal fluid cannot enter this second barrier. During sleep, the neural cells relax and allow cerebrospinal fluid to flow through brain's cells to help replenish it.[22]

While this is happening, your body's main obligation to your brain is to make sure it's getting enough oxygen. If the supply of oxygen is compromised or interrupted, it can lead to serious health problems.

According to the National Institutes of Health, up to 70 million Americans are affected by chronic sleep disorders.[23] Most people wouldn't think they're at risk, but what they don't realize is that anyone who hasn't had proper dental, jaw, or facial development *is* at risk.

You probably know someone who snores. There's a good chance you've snored yourself. For the most part, we view it as an annoying quirk—or, if it doesn't keep us up at night, a funny one. But the truth is that snoring is linked to some very serious illnesses, including heart disease and mental degeneration.

What causes snoring?

If you're asleep and your airways are too narrow or obstructed, you might snore. Snoring is the sound of tissues in those airways vibrating due to the blockage as you breathe in and out.

If your jaw is underdeveloped—which often leads to impacted wisdom teeth or crooked teeth—there's less space inside your mouth. That means there's less space for your tongue. As a result, it can fall back inside your mouth when you lie down, block your airway, interrupt your breathing, and cause you to snore.

If you snore . . .

In The Dental Diet program, we will include exercises to help improve your breathing. Retraining your daytime breathing may help your breathing at night. Staying active by exercising helps too. It might take some time, but training yourself to breathe through your nose may also help. If you can get to the point where you breathe through your nose during the night out of habit, you'll snore less and give your body more oxygen in the process.

The medical term for snoring is sleep apnea. (Technically, an apnea is a temporary stoppage in breathing that usually happens during sleep). An apnea can be caused when your upper airway is obstructed or when your brain isn't getting the right signals to the muscles that control your breathing.[24]

In a severe apnea, the consistent interruption to breathing can disrupt the flow of oxygen to the brain and damage the parts that regulate brain pressure and heart rate. This can lead to serious issues like dementia and heart disease.[25] So while snoring may seem harmless, it's important to realize that its long-term consequences can be severe.

It's estimated that 25 million Americans suffer from obstructive sleep apnea, or OSA.[26] The main risk factors include age, weight, and craniofacial anatomy—the shape of your skull and face.[27] And that's where jaw development comes in.

What sleep apnea can do to your brain

Brain scans of people with sleep apnea reveal that when we don't sleep at night, important parts of the brain suffer damage.[28,29] These include parts of the brain that help regulate the autonomic nervous system, which controls the unconscious processes in our body. Specifically, sleep apnea has been shown to harm the regions that influence breathing, blood pressure and motor coordination, and memories, including memories of smells.

The hippocampus is the part of the brain that controls short and long-term memory as well as spatial memory. It is the first to be damaged in Alzheimer's disease and can be found to be damaged in OSA. Exercise can help the hippocampus to regenerate neurons. That's why physical activity is an important part of any treatment for a breathing-related disorder.

Teeth grinding syndrome

For a long time in my practice, I noticed many patients—usually in their twenties and usually women—who suffered from digestive problems like constipation, bloating, and irritable bowel syndrome, along with cold hands and feet, anxiety, and/or depression. They often had worn-out, flattened teeth that told me they were nighttime teeth grinders. What did all of these people have in common? Small jaws that didn't support their airways.

For many years, dentists would prescribe a splint to stop the damage to their teeth. What no one realized, however, was that these women had a worse problem than worn teeth. They were showing telltale signs of sleep-disordered breathing.

We used to think that sleep apnea was confined to overweight and elderly males. But now we know that it has a little sister, called upper airway resistance syndrome (UARS), that impacts a much larger group of people. A relatively new classification of breathing disorders, it wasn't discovered until 1993, when it was identified by researchers at Stanford.[30]

People who suffer from UARS have airways that collapse more easily due to their smaller mouths and jaws. As a result, they're constantly in a state of interrupted sleep, during which their brain is being told that their airway needs to be opened (much like the choking response). This activates the sympathetic nervous system—the body's survival mode—which releases adrenaline and sends the body into constant stress. This often causes the jaw to be pushed forward and results in the grinding of teeth.

The sympathetic nervous system also turns off the digestive system and sends blood to the rest of the body, which explains the digestive issues associated with those who suffer from UARS—the same symptoms experienced by the women I saw in my practice.

Dr. Steven Y. Park, M D, a New York ear, nose, and throat surgeon and author of Sleep Interrupted describes UARS patients very well:

> All UARS patients have some form of fatigue, almost all state that they are "light sleepers," and almost invariably, they don't like to sleep on their backs. In some cases, they actually can't. Some people attribute their poor-quality sleep to insomnia, stress, or working too much. Due to repetitive arousals at night, especially during the deeper levels of sleep, one is unable to get the required deep, restorative sleep that one needs to feel refreshed in the morning. In most cases, the anatomic reason for this collapse is the tongue. There are many reasons for the tongue to cause obstruction, including being too large or being overweight. But once it occurs, the only thing you can do is to wake up.[31]

For a long time, I saw patients with typical symptoms of UARS. Eventually I realized they all had something in common: small mouths and jaws with or without previous orthodontia.

Symptoms of UARS include:

- Digestive issues like irritable bowel syndrome (IBD), Crohn's disease, chronic diarrhea, constipation, indigestion, acid reflux, or bloating.[32]

- Cold feet and hands. (Some people have Raynaud's phenomenon, a condition where the blood vessels in the fingers and toes narrow, slowing circulation; many have to wear gloves year-round.)

- Low blood pressure, dizziness, and light-headedness called orthostatic intolerance (23 percent of people with UARS have low blood pressure).[33]

- Chronic runny or stuffy nose

- Sinus pain, sinus headaches, migraines, tension headaches

- Stress, teeth clenching, depression, anxiety (or ADHD in children)[34]

- Teeth grinding[35]

These symptoms are bad enough, but the bigger problem is that a person in their twenties with UARS may turn into a person in their forties who snores and has a higher risk of sleep apnea as well as brain and heart conditions.

We are now beginning to retrain people who have breathing disorders *how* to breathe. I describe some of these breathing exercises at the end of this chapter, but throughout the Dental Diet program you'll learn exercises to retrain your breathing to get more oxygen.

Childhood behavior disorders, sleep disorders, mouth breathing, and ADHD

Crooked teeth, which are an epidemic among children, are a sign that a person's jaw hasn't developed properly and that their airways are likely cramped and small. So it shouldn't come as a surprise that close to one-third of all kids suffer from sleep disorders, which tend to begin as breathing disorders. In certain populations, including children with special needs and those with psychiatric or medical conditions, the rate of sleep disorders is even higher.[36]

The most common symptoms I see in the kids with crooked teeth who come to my practice are venous pooling under the eyes, cracked and dry lips, poor head posture, bed-wetting, poor school results, constant tiredness, and an open mouth at rest.

They have a hard time getting up in the morning, even after a long night of sleep. They snore, grind their teeth, suffer from headaches, have trouble concentrating, and are either prone to aggression or generally "cranky."

We need to understand that all of these disordered breathing conditions, including sleep apnea and UARS, are craniofacial growth problems. When the jaw, teeth, and face don't develop the way they should during childhood, the airways don't function as they're meant to throughout life. This can lead to sleep apnea and, if that's not treated, heart failure and brain degeneration later on.

Signs of normal and poor facial development

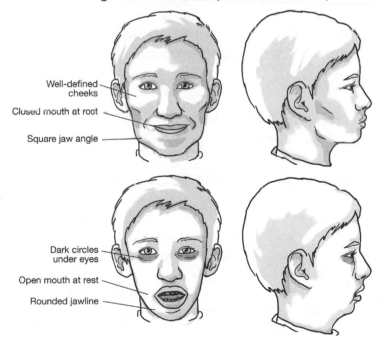

Well-defined cheeks
Closed mouth at rest
Square jaw angle

Dark circles under eyes
Open mouth at rest
Rounded jawline

Fig. 9. Facial development and mouth breathing in children

Does apnea lead to ADHD in children?

Around 25 percent of all children experience some type of sleep problem, and around 12 percent present snoring and sleep apnea.[37] In contrast, sleep complaints in children with ADHD have been reported in 55 percent of cases.[38] Children undergoing evaluation for ADHD should routinely be screened for sleep disorders.

A lack of sleep can damage brain neurons, particularly in the prefrontal cortex region. This may be due to a decrease in oxygen and an increase in carbon dioxide levels, interference with sleep's restorative processes, and a disruption in the balance of cellular and chemical systems. Inattentiveness, hyperactivity, and impulsivity—the classic trademarks of ADHD—can result.

If there is a misdiagnosis of ADHD, this can be problematic when one considers the fact that medications used to treat ADHD, like Ritalin, are stimulants and can cause insomnia. In some countries, a child cannot be prescribed medication for ADHD until their breathing at night has been assessed. Suffice it to say, snoring is not harmless in kids.

FUNCTIONAL TREATMENTS FOR SLEEP APNEA

While the disorders above are serious health issues, there are effective things you can do to strengthen your airway muscles, which will fight off these disorders if you have them and protect you from getting them if you don't. It's all about correcting one of the most ingrained behaviors you have—your breathing habits.

We know that exercise itself is beneficial for the cerebellum, which is one of the areas of the brain that suffers damage during sleep apnea.[39] Interestingly, studies have shown that taking up the Australian didgeridoo can help fight off sleep apnea as well.[40] Playing the ancient instrument is known to exercise and strengthen the airways. Or you could take opera classes. Singing opera strengthens the airway muscles and retrains the brain to use them. Even performing some simple daily tongue exercises helps to improve your breathing.

Breathing, voice, and tongue exercises are all part of keeping your jaw and teeth functioning as they should. However, another important factor is eating whole, collagenous, fibrous foods that require your jaw muscles to chew. (The trick is that you have to primarily use your mastication, or chewing, muscles, not your facial muscles.)

EXERCISES TO CORRECT YOUR BREATHING

First you need to reprogram yourself to breathe through your nose, if you don't already. You'll be astounded by the benefits of consciously making sure you breathe through your nose during the day and night. (People with developmental issues may need to see an ear, nose, and throat specialist to see if they have a restriction that is preventing nasal breathing.)

You can also help yourself breathe better by improving the functional habits of your mouth and jaw. The following exercises will help.

Diaphragmatic breathing exercise (three minutes per day)

Slower, deeper breathing allows your body to extract more oxygen from the air. It also activates your parasympathetic nervous system, which helps your digestive system to function at its peak.

This exercise is designed to help you use your diaphragmatic muscles when you breathe in. Your belly should expand instead of your chest. (When you breathe into your belly by contracting your diaphragm it maximizes the space for your lungs to expand to and take in air.)

1. Sit with your back straight and your mouth closed. Put one hand over your belly and relax your shoulders, jaw, and neck.
2. Breathe in for 3 seconds, letting your belly expand. When you inhale, you should feel your hand being pushed forward by the expansion of your belly.
3. Release the air through your nose, slowly (4 seconds). Picture that you are letting air out gently and slowly through a thin straw.
4. Your hand should move back toward you as you pull your belly back toward your spine. Once your hand stops moving, pause for 1 to 2 seconds, then inhale again.
5. Repeat the cycle 20 times (3 seconds in, 4 seconds out).

If you have trouble, keep practicing. It takes time to learn to use these muscle groups to breathe this way.

Tongue exercise (three minutes, twice a day)

This exercise will help hold your tongue at the top of your mouth while you rest, which will help the muscles stay active at night.

Hold your tongue behind your back teeth, just behind the two grooves on your palate. Push upward, including the sides and back of your tongue, to the roof of the mouth, and hold for three minutes. Do this twice a day.

Voice exercise

Exercise your voice and throat muscles by humming (think of the "ohm" performed in yoga).

1. Keep your eyes closed and take a deep breath into your diaphragm for 3 seconds. Then let out a quiet hum—it should be deep, but everyone's will be different. Picture the hum starting in your stomach and moving like a violin bow over your vocal cords. Do this for 2 minutes.

2. Then point your tongue to your palate. You should notice the hum getting slightly higher, and your upper jaw should vibrate. Hum into your upper jaw like that for another 2 minutes.

CHAPTER 4

THE MYSTERY OF THE MISSING VITAMIN

THE TOOTH CARE PARADOX

I see it all the time in my practice.

Young siblings come in for a checkup with the same brushing habits, but one kid has multiple cavities while the other has spotless, healthy teeth. And it doesn't just happen with kids; I see it with adults, too (although they don't usually come in at the same time).

Maybe you've had a similar experience, if not with a relative, then with a friend. You take great pains to take care of your teeth—you always brush, you floss regularly—while your friend does these things erratically and half-heartedly at best. But every time you go to the dentist, you need a lot of work on your mouth, while your friend is always in and out with very little fuss. Or maybe you and your friend take similar care of your teeth, but you still have very different diagnoses from the dentist.

There's no way around it. Some people seem immune to tooth decay, and some people seem prone to it no matter what they do. They endure the painful dentist visits, year after year, by resigning themselves to the idea that they have "weak enamel" or just "weak teeth."

They're not wrong, actually. But they're right for the wrong reasons. Obviously when two people experience different states of oral health and the difference can't be explained by their personal hygiene habits, something about their teeth *is* different. But this difference isn't genetic—at least, not as much as you may think.

Instead, there's a good chance that one person's teeth are stronger because of their diet. In other words, that person probably eats more of the foods that have the nutrients their teeth need to fight off disease and decay.

A lot of people think that their teeth are basically inanimate objects that they have to take care of from the outside—like ceramic vases that they need to clean and polish but that can't maintain themselves. But nothing could be further from the truth. Our teeth are very much alive on the inside, and they need a very specific balance of minerals, vitamins, and proteins to stay strong and healthy.

In fact, just as our bones have marrow and other cells that build and maintain our skeletal system, our teeth have living inner cores that essentially make them functioning organs unto themselves. If you want a healthy mouth, you have to treat them right. And as it turns out, this will keep the rest of your body healthy, too.

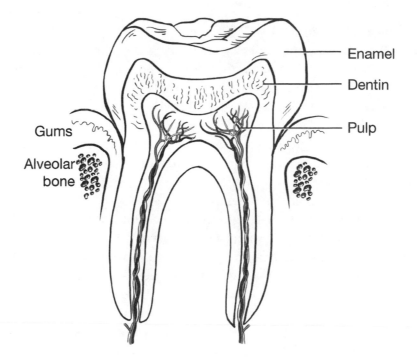

Enamel

Dentin

Pulp

Gums

Alveolar bone

Fig. 10. What the inside of a tooth looks like

As you can see in this diagram, each of our teeth has a thick sheet of enamel on the outside—that's the part we see, and it is, for all intents and purposes, inanimate. After our tooth enamel is fully formed, it's the hardest substance in our body, comprising a higher percentage of minerals than anything else we produce. But enamel is not made up of living cells, so if it cracks or deteriorates, the body is unable to repair it.

By the same token, enamel doesn't have its own immune system. It's at the mercy of the elements—the saliva, minerals, and food as well as the bacteria, the plaque they build, acids, and other substances that pass through our mouths every day. Our tooth enamel has to endure this hostile, ever-changing mix of substances, along with the incredible pressure and friction we subject it to as we chew our food. (And the truth is, we don't just expect our enamel to endure—we expect it to look as white and shiny as polished ivory.)

Sounds like our enamel is in a pretty tough spot, right? Fortunately, it has a couple of big allies to help protect it against decay. They're the two inner layers of the tooth: the dentin and the pulp.

The dentin is the layer of tissue that serves as a sort of insulation beneath the enamel, and the pulp is the inner core of the tooth. The pulp is the life-support system of the tooth. It connects it to the nervous system, which monitors how the tooth is doing, and to the blood supply, which gives the tooth the resources it needs for growth and maintenance.

The dentin is the battleground of the tooth. It's the dentin's job to make sure that the chaos that swirls inside the mouth doesn't make its way near the precious pulp. So it houses a team of cells, kind of like a SWAT team, that seeks out and eliminates unwanted microbes that make their way through the enamel.[1]

Where do these cells come from? Well, the cells that fight foreign invaders in your teeth are the very same cells that build your teeth in the first place. And they're similar to the cells that make your bones.

Your bone marrow produces stem cells that eventually mature into different cells that play different roles in your body. These stem cells get signals (hormones sent from the endocrine system) that tell them whether to become bone-making cells, teeth-making cells, immune cells, red blood cells, or platelets.[2] It's all part of the osteoimmunity system, where the skeletal and immune systems and the minerals they need to function are all maintained in delicate balance.[3] And there's no better example of it in action than inside each and every one of your teeth.

Whereas marrow produces osteoblasts and osteoclasts (the worker cells that build and maintain bone), teeth have cells that build and maintain dentin, called odontoblasts. But odontoblasts aren't just builders. They're also the guards of the dentin and pulp—they release immune cells that fight infectious bacteria that make it through the bony maze of enamel. And, if the dentin does suffer damage, the odontoblasts work to patch it up so that the invading microbes don't reach the pulp.[4]

Evidence that our teeth build, protect, and repair themselves from the inside can be found in the fact that teeth that have lost their blood and nerve supply develop decay much faster than living teeth.[5] These "dead" teeth are the ones that require root canal treatment.

You can't just take care of your teeth from the outside; you have to protect what's inside of them as well. Far from inanimate objects, your teeth are constantly building, maintaining, and protecting themselves from the outside world.

VITAMIN D: THE CEO OF YOUR BONES, TEETH, AND IMMUNE CELLS

You might say that odontoblasts have a pretty important job to do, and you'd be right. But if you want a job done well, you need to give whoever's doing it the right tools, and odontoblasts are no exception.

To do their job well, odontoblasts need a vitamin that your entire body should get every day: vitamin D.[6] You probably know that your body needs vitamin D to keep your bones strong and healthy. Your odontoblasts also need it to keep your teeth healthy.

Vitamin D is one of the major factors that determine whether the stem cells from your bone marrow grow and mature into bone-forming cells, blood cells, or immune cells. It also regulates how all of these cells operate. For instance, vitamin D can produce immune cells that make specific antibodies (B-cells),[7] but it can also slow the release of immune cells that can cause inflammation if they build up too much.[8]

In animal studies, a lack of vitamin D has been shown to disrupt dentin formation.[9] So if you want your teeth's immunity specialists to keep a constant watch over your teeth, you need to give them enough vitamin D. Low vitamin D has been linked to risk of tooth decay in children[10] and gum disease in adults.[11]

But vitamin D does far more than manage the immune system inside the tooth. It also helps supply our bones, teeth, and muscles with the raw material, the "cement," they need most to build themselves up: calcium. Vitamin D helps the intestines to absorb calcium from the foods we eat, and, like a delivery truck, it helps carry it through the bloodstream to the rest of the body. In fact, if you ate food rich in calcium but your body didn't have enough vitamin D, it would absorb only 10 to 15 percent of the calcium you took in.[12]

Calcium is used in many cellular processes throughout the body, including the contraction of muscles. Accordingly, when your body is low on vitamin D, and hence calcium, it releases a hormone called parathyroid hormone that forces your bones and teeth to release calcium[13] so it can be used for things like muscle contraction. Calcium is a precious commodity to your body, and it's up to vitamin D to make sure it's used efficiently.

But vitamin D does even more than regulate stem cells and help your body use calcium. In fact, if oxygen is the most important nutrient for your body, vitamin D runs a close second. Between 2,000 and 3,000 genes in the body have receptors for vitamin D,[14] and it plays a central role in countless physiological processes:

- It controls hormones and cell growth.
- It regulates digestion and gut microbes.
- It helps with balance.
- It influences metabolism.
- It strengthens the body against respiratory infections, cancer, heart disease, diabetes, and other ailments.
- It aids neurological function.[15]

There's even evidence that vitamin D helps prevent colon, breast, prostate, and ovarian cancers,[16] Alzheimer's disease,[17] and multiple sclerosis[18] and that it slows aging.[19] Low vitamin D has been linked to obesity[20] as well as a range of digestive disorders, like irritable bowel syndrome (IBS)[21] celiac disease,[22] ulcerative colitis,[23] and Crohn's disease.[24]

For the most part, our skin synthesizes vitamin D from ultraviolet radiation in the sun's rays. But most of us probably don't get quite enough of it, so I always recommend that my patients get more sunlight. But if you just *can't* get enough sunlight, or your body has trouble synthesizing it (which is common), you need to get vitamin D through your diet, which is a bit tricky because it's found only in certain foods.

Even so, vitamin D alone isn't enough to keep your teeth, bones, and body completely healthy. Vitamin D has its own support team that it needs to keep your body working like a finely tuned watch.

The calcium paradox

Dentists see calcified plaque all the time. We spend a good amount of time scraping it off of our patients' teeth. To prevent problems with plaque, our main advice is to brush and floss regularly. But I've found that many people with good oral hygiene still get heavy calculus (calcified dental plaque) buildup, while others barely get any despite not brushing all. This is because heavy dental calculus is as much a sign that the body can't put minerals where they need to go as it is an indicator of oral hygiene.

Let's look at what this means in the rest of the body.

Osteoporosis is a disease where a person's bones become weak and brittle, and can easily break. It affects about 50 percent of adults over the age of 65, and some figures suggest up to 80 percent of older adults are affected.[25]

As we've said, the mineral calcium is sort of like a cement our body uses to build and strengthen our teeth and bones, and vitamin D is like a truck that delivers the calcium where it's needed. For a long time, older women at risk of osteoporosis were prescribed calcium and vitamin D supplements. The thinking was that, if bones naturally become weaker as we age, giving these women extra calcium and vitamin D would make it easier for their bodies to keep their bones strong and healthy.

But it didn't pan out that way. A paper published in 2011 showed that, surprisingly, women who took these supplements didn't experience much improvement in bone density. Not only that, but the supplements *increased* their risk of heart disease.[26]

Researchers were stumped by these results. If the body needs calcium and vitamin D to maintain strong, healthy bones, why would consuming *extra* quantities of calcium and vitamin D do so little for bones and even harm other organs?

ON THE HUNT FOR ACTIVATOR X

Earlier we discussed the research of Dr. Weston Price. Throughout Price's work, he referred to a mysterious "vitamin-like activator" that helped the body use minerals and fight tooth decay and allowed people to grow strong, healthy jaws. Dubbing it "Activator X," Price demonstrated that it worked with two other "fat-soluble activators," vitamins A and D.

In his laboratory, by studying nutrients from food samples he had taken from the traditional cultures, Price was able to prove that Activator X *existed*. But he never uncovered its chemical structure.

It turned out that Activator X was the fat-soluble vitamin K2. But no one would discover that until decades later. Reviewing that discovery is important because it shows us why K2 is *still* relatively unknown and why our modern diet doesn't give us enough of it.

What *is* a vitamin, anyway?

A vitamin is a nutrient (technically an organic compound) that your body needs small amounts of to function properly. Organisms need a range of vitamins; they synthesize (make) some of these themselves, and they obtain others from the environment, meaning they need to get them through their diet. In fact, there are vitamins that some animals can synthesize on their own while other species have to get them through food. For example, humans need ascorbic acid, a form of vitamin C, to prevent scurvy. Since ascorbic acid is derived from glucose (sugar), many animals can produce it on their own, but humans cannot.

The word *vitamin* was coined in 1912 by Polish biochemist Casimir Funk.[27] It comes from a compound word, *vitamine*, that combines *vital* and *amine*. Amines are compounds that have a basic nitrogen atom with a "free" pair of electrons. In 1912, it was thought that all compounds that fit the definition of *vitamin* might be amines. Thiamine, or vitamin B, is an amine, but it turned out that none of the others were. *Vitamine* was then shortened to *vitamin* in English.

There are no vitamins between E and K because the compounds originally given those letters have either been reclassified or proven to be false leads.

While we're here, what's a fat-soluble vitamin?

Vitamins are classified as either water-soluble or fat-soluble. For people, there are 13 vitamins: 4 are fat-soluble (A, D, E, and K) and 9 are water-soluble (eight B vitamins and vitamin C). Water-soluble vitamins dissolve best in water and tend to be excreted from the body more easily, through the kidneys and eventually the urine.

The word "vitamin" may be a bit misleading for some of the fat-soluble vitamins. Technically, vitamin D isn't a vitamin. It's actually a prohormone that's produced photochemically (through the chemical action of light). The molecular structure of vitamin D is close to that of classic steroid hormones, and vitamin D plays roles that are similar to those of steroids.

One last thing—what do we mean by activate?

When we say that a vitamin "activates" a protein or that one compound is an "activator" for another, it means that the vitamin chemically alters the protein when it interacts with it. It switches it to its active form, something the body can use.

The discovery of vitamin K1 and K2, and their roles in the body

In the early 1930s, Danish biochemist Henrik Dam discovered a compound that helped blood to clot. In 1935 he published a paper in a German journal that introduced this substance as vitamin K, named after the German word for coagulation (*koagulation*).[28] He described the compound wholly as "vitamin K," but noted that it had two chemical forms, in K1 and K2. K2 was said to have molecular structure that is close to, but not quite the same as, that of K1. But since the molecular structures of K1 and K2 were so similar, he assumed they served the same function in blood clotting[29,30] and lumped them under the same name, vitamin K.*

As it turns out, K1 mainly helps with blood clotting, while K2 mainly serves to activate two proteins, osteocalcin[31] and matrix GLA-protein (MGP),[32] which make sure calcium goes where it's supposed to—into bones and teeth, and not into arteries.[33] But no one connected those dots until decades later.

The big reveal: How Activator X was identified as vitamin K2

One day in 2005, Sally Fallon Morell, co-founder of the Weston A. Price Foundation, got an e-mail from Michael Eiseike, a health researcher from Hokkaido, Japan, who recommended that she look into a study that had just come out of Rotterdam. "I think this might be Activator X," he wrote.

The study showed that vitamin K2 was associated with a 52 percent lower risk of severe aortic calcification, a 41 percent lower risk of coronary heart disease (CHD), a 51 percent lower risk of CHD mortality, and a 26 percent lower risk of total mortality."[34] Those findings seemed to echo Price's assertion that Activator X was a crucial factor in how the body prevents heart disease, among other things.

---

* You may wonder why, if vitamins K1 and K2 have different chemical structures, people didn't assume they have different purposes as well. But this sort of thing happens all the time in biology. For example, think about the pigmentation of your eyes. Your genes determine whether your eyes are brown, blue, or green, and if you had slightly different genes, they'd be a different color. But no matter the color of your eyes, their pigmentation would play the same role: protecting your retinas from the sun.

Fallon e-mailed Chris Masterjohn, an assistant professor of health and nutrition sciences at Brooklyn College and one of the most recognized experts on fat-soluble vitamins in the world. She told him about Eiseike's theory and the study on K2. Masterjohn did some more digging.

The more he dug, the more evidence Masterjohn found that Activator X could indeed be K2. For instance, he found a 2004 study from Japan that said that K2 "reversed bone loss in the elderly and sometimes even increased bone mass in people with osteoporosis."[35] Seven other Japanese studies collectively showed that K2 led to a "60 percent reduction in vertebral fractures and 80 percent reduction in hip and other non-vertebral fractures."[36] Those studies paralleled Price's claim that Activator X was a crucial factor in bone growth and maintenance, as well as other factors.

But for Masterjohn, "the lightbulb really went off" when he discovered that vitamin K1 is found in large quantities in chlorophyll, which plays a key role in photosynthesis, the process by which plants convert light to energy so they can grow. As Masterjohn learned, when cows eat grass that has vitamin K1 in it, they convert it to K2 in their tissue. The more K1 there is in the grass, the more K2 there is in the cows, and the more K2 there is in the butter produced from their milk. Price had said that Activator X was found in higher quantities in places whose inhabitants harvested fast-growing spring grass, which we now know contains more vitamin K1.

Now the parallels between what Price said about Activator X and what Chris learned about K2 were too strong to deny. He finally responded to Fallon's e-mail regarding Eiseike's belief that Activator X was K2.

"I think he's right," he said.

Masterjohn sums this up in his article "On the Trail of the Elusive X-Factor: A Sixty-Two-Year-Old Mystery Finally Solved."[37]

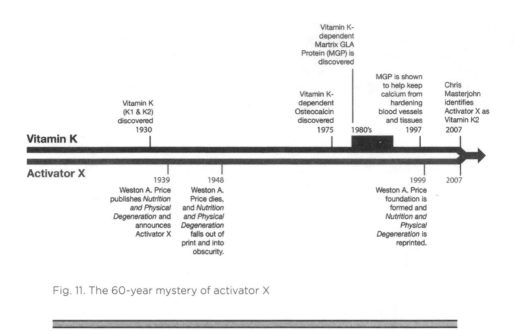

Fig. 11. The 60-year mystery of activator X

YOUR TEETH AND BODY DEPEND ON VITAMIN K2

We now know that vitamin K2 plays a role in forming and strengthening bones by activating osteocalcin, which helps carry calcium *into* bones.[38] We also know that K2 activates Matrix GLA Protein, which helps *remove* calcium from arteries to prevent artery hardening.[39]

This explains why a shortage of vitamin K2 would prevent the women in the 2011 study that we talked about earlier from getting stronger bones from calcium and vitamin D supplements. Without the K2 to activate the proteins that carry calcium, the body can't place calcium where it is supposed to go.[40] It also explains why some of them suffered from heart disease.

K2 also prevents the calcium deposition responsible for kidney stones[41] and is considered a crucial marker in the progression of kidney disease.[42] Studies are also showing its role in preventing the formation of gallstones[43] and in protecting men from prostate cancer.[44]

So the next time you see calculus buildup on your teeth, you might consider how this may be happening in the vessels throughout your body. By understanding what K2 does in the body, you can see how the same process that calcifies arteries also calcifies the plaque on our teeth, and why dietary analyses inevitably reveal that people with dental calculus don't eat enough foods rich in vitamin K2.

Because we only recently learned how it works, we still don't have reliable tests to measure vitamin K2 in the body. You won't see K2 in the nutritional information on food packages either. However, we do know which foods tend to be higher in K2.

When animals consume vitamin K1, which is found not only in grass but in green leafy vegetables, their digestive system converts it to K2. (Yet another reason why grass-fed animals produce healthier meat than grain-fed animals.) There are two types of vitamin K2, the animal-derived MK-4 and the bacteria-derived MK-7. Good sources of K2 (MK-4 form) include organ meats, eggs from pasture-raised chickens, butter from grass-fed cows, shellfish, and emu oil.

K2 (MK-7 form) can also be created by the fermentation of bacteria, so foods like Japanese natto (a fermented soybean), sauerkraut, and cheeses like Gouda and brie are also good sources.

Vitamin K2 and facial growth

If you don't breathe mainly through your nose, your jaw and teeth won't grow the way they should. But if your body doesn't have the raw materials to properly build the airways that *let* you breathe through your nose, are your jaw and teeth doomed from the outset?

This could be the case for people with deviated nasal septa, which might be caused by a lack of K2.

Is K2 the culprit behind deviated septa?

Without K2, calcium doesn't go into bones, but instead goes into the soft tissue. In the skull, this may cause the nasal septum (cartilage) to calcify, which stops its growth. This underdeveloped nasal cartilage may lead to a deviated septum—a septum that is misaligned with the nostrils and airways of the nose—or other facial deformities.

Studies have been done on vitamin K-deficient rats whose septal cartilage became calcified. These rats developed unusual faces that had extremely truncated snouts. The prevailing theory behind this phenomenon is that the nose and middle of the face can develop properly only when the septal cartilage remains elastic. If it hardens, it locks the face into an underdeveloped or malformed framework.[45]

Today, deviated septa are quite common. Some studies estimate that as many as 80 percent of the population have them.[46] These people's faces might not look underdeveloped on the outside, but it's quite possible that their deviated septa are a sign of underdeveloped bones and airways on the inside.

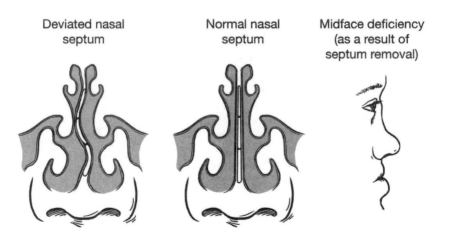

Fig. 12. Deviated nasal septum, facial shape, and development

VITAMIN A—THE *FINAL* PUZZLE PIECE?

There's one more piece to our puzzle of tooth and bone development: vitamin A. While its role the body is not completely understood, we know that vitamin A is crucial for fetal development[47] and eyesight.[48]

Vitamin A comprises a group of organic compounds including retinol, retinal, retinoic acid, and beta-carotene.[49] We know that it plays a key role in helping teeth and bones develop, in reproduction, and in regulating the immune system.[50] And it helps the membranes of our skin, eyes, mouth, nose, throat, and lungs to stay moist.

While we don't fully understand how vitamin A contributes to bone development, it seems that it helps cells called osteoclasts that break down bone.[51] During bone growth, the bone must remain functional. In order to grow new bone cells, the existing cells need to be "broken down." Once osteoclasts do their job, osteoblasts can come in and properly lay down new bone tissue. Vitamin A seems to drive this by kicking osteoclasts into action.

Plants and microorganisms make their own vitamin A. But animals that are higher up on the food chain, like humans, have to get it from their diet. Animal foods are better sources of the active form of vitamin A than plant foods, and cod-liver oil is a particularly good source.

Is vitamin A the culprit behind cleft palate?

As a human fetus develops in the womb, its brain and spinal cord grow out of an embryonic structure called the neural tube. As the spinal cord is completed in the bony case of the vertebrae, the body goes through a set of "checkpoints." At each of these, it must end its current work and move to the next developmental stage. As the weeks pass, a fetus passes through many of these "checkpoints" that usually occur after a set period of time. Vitamin B12 is one of the crucial nutrients the body uses to form neural and brain tissue. If there is inadequate B12 available and the checkpoint is reached, the body must move on, even if development is incomplete.

An example of this is spina bifida, where the neural tube has failed to close up and part of the spinal cord can bulge out from the vertebrae. Studies have linked this condition to a lack of vitamin B12.[52] The body reaches its checkpoint with an unfinished spinal cord, but the show must move on.

The physiological process of a cleft palate and lip (where the roof of the mouth fails to close properly) is similar to the developmental problem in children suffering from spina bifida. In a healthy baby, the neural tube zips all the way up the spine and through the palate, ending at the upper lip.

It's not fully understood which factors lead to cleft palates and lips. But a 2011 study showed that babies born with cleft palates also tend to have significant developmental problems with their eyes.[53] This is reminiscent of vitamin A deficiency. Fred Hale, an animal husbandry and swine nutrition specialist from the Texas Agricultural Experiment Station, performed Vitamin A experiments on pigs in the 1930s. When pigs were stripped of vitamin A, they developed cleft palates on top of severe eye problems.[54]

The cause of cleft palates in humans may be linked to a lack of vitamin A and the role vitamin A plays in facial and bone development along with vitamins D and K2.

HOW THE PIECES ALL FIT TOGETHER

Now that we've completed our puzzle (at least for the time being), let's go over why the pieces are so important for your health.

Vitamins A and D essentially tell our cells to produce certain proteins—osteocalcin and MGP—that help build and repair teeth and bones by taking calcium where it needs to go, among other things. But for the body to use these proteins, it has to call on vitamin K2 to activate them.

If you're thinking it's all bit complicated and hard to grasp, you're not alone. Think about how long it took the scientific community as a whole to get to the bottom of these processes. To help you understand what we *do* know, remember our analogy in which vitamin D is a truck that delivers cement through your body so the right cells can use it to build up the right structures.

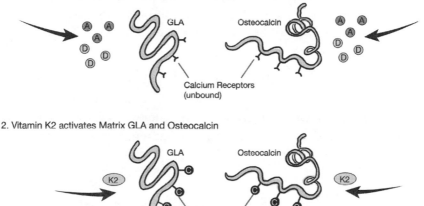

1. Vitamin A and Vitamin D synthesize Matrix GLA protein and Osteocalcin

2. Vitamin K2 activates Matrix GLA and Osteocalcin

Fig. 13. The synergistic role of vitamins A, D, and K2 in placing calcium into bones and teeth

Let's flesh it out even more:

- Vitamin D is the cement (calcium) delivery truck.

- Vitamin A is the scaffolding and workers.

- Osteocalcin and MGP protein are like quality controls. They make sure the cement gets to the right building projects and doesn't clog up the water, electrical, and other moving systems.

- Vitamin K2 turns the cement mixer on and activates the concrete.

- Without K2, the workers just drop wet, unset concrete onto the building walls (bone). It falls off and clumps up where it shouldn't.

- If this goes on, there's eventually unset concrete everywhere on the building site and in the plumbing and the generator (or in our case, our arteries and organs), where it clogs up and shuts the system down.

In this way, vitamins K2, A, and D play key roles in how our facial bones develop. Each is crucial in its own respect and all require the actions of the others. And they work in this amazing symphony to direct the tiny immune system inside your teeth.

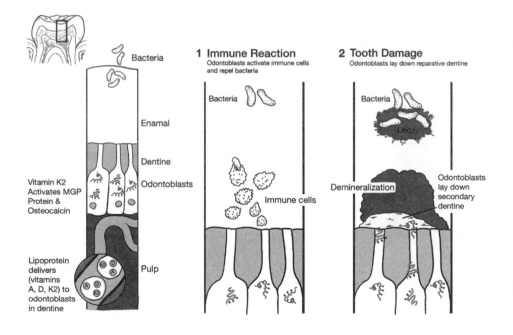

Fig. 14. How Vitamins A, D, and K2 activate the immune system inside your teeth

THE SECRET TO HEALTH THAT'S HIDDEN IN YOUR TEETH

One of the amazing things about traditional diets around the world is that, generally, they were meticulously focused on providing adequate amounts of vitamins A, D, and K2 even before we had names for these nutrients.

Along those lines, one of the major differences between our modern diet and traditional diets is that the food we eat doesn't give us enough of these vitamins. So the immune system inside our teeth just doesn't have what it needs to do its job. And no matter how well we take care of our teeth from the outside, we often can't avoid tooth decay unless we radically change how we eat.

That's why the Dental Diet focuses on foods that are rich in fat-soluble vitamins—to give your mouth the tools it might not have gotten enough of for your entire life. And the beauty of this is that these same foods are rich in the other nutrients your mouth and body need as well.

CHAPTER 5

THE LANGUAGE OF BACTERIA

How Your Mouth Controls Your Gut

As a dentist, when I talk to patients about "sweets," the response is almost always the same. There is a sheepish admission that they have a sweet tooth, and yes, they know that by eating a lot of sugar, they're putting themselves at risk for tooth decay. Even young kids understand the relationship between sugar and tooth decay, a trade-off they're normally more than happy to make.

I think the main reason people are so cavalier about sugar and decay is that they figure the worst that can happen is that they'll get a cavity, the dentist will fill it, and they'll be back to normal in no time.

But what most people don't realize is that when you get a cavity, it's more than a sign that you're consuming too many sugary foods and drinks; it's a sign that some important processes in your *body* aren't working properly—processes you might not even know exist. In this chapter, we're going to look closely at them and learn what we can do to get them back up to speed.

But first, let's do a little thought experiment. I'm going to give you a word, and I want you to take a moment to think about how it makes you feel and what you associate with it.

The word is: *bacteria*.

What does that make you think about? I'm guessing it's things like disease, or germs, or filth, and you may be reaching for your antibacterial hand sanitizer right now. That's fair. Bacteria *are* a key factor in all of those negative things. In fact, they're a huge player in tooth decay, too.

For a long time, we took it for granted that tooth decay was mainly caused by poor oral hygiene (which allows bacteria to grow in the mouth) and eating too much sugar (which, when consumed by bacteria, creates acid and then decay). Here's a simple way of describing the relationship:

Sugar + Bacteria = Acid
Acid + Tooth = Dental Decay

Unquestionably, these two statements are true, but they're missing many of the connecting dots that explain *how* bacteria and sugar can create decay when they combine. Nor do they explain why some people can eat a lot of sugar and get relatively little decay, while others are constantly fighting decay no matter how much they brush and floss.

This is because we've only recently begun to understand bacteria's complex role in the mouth and body.

In the past several years, we've learned that our whole body is actually filled with bacteria that it needs to stay *healthy*. And the mouth and teeth are no exception. Our mouth is in a permanent partnership with bacteria that help maintain our teeth and gums and also our mouth's immune system. Tooth decay is a sign that the bacteria in the mouth are imbalanced, and it can also be a sign of trouble in the rest of the body.

To understand why this is, we have to gain a better appreciation for everything bacteria do to help us stay healthy and why we've misunderstood their many important roles for so long.

A SHORT HISTORY OF THE WAR ON MICROBES

How did bacteria get such a bad reputation in the first place? The answer basically boils down to human error.

Today we take it for granted that there's microscopic life all around us—and *in* us. But for most of human history, people didn't know it was there. They suspected there was something out there causing diseases, and that "bad air" arose from decaying matter, but that was about it. During times of plague, doctors wore elaborate masks with beaks full of herbs that they believed would keep foul vapors from entering their bodies.

In 1674, Dutch tradesman and amateur lens maker Antonie van Leeuwenhoek created a microscope that was much more powerful than anything that had come before it.[1] With this newfound power of magnification, van Leeuwenhoek discovered that there were virtually invisible organisms living everywhere. He dubbed them "animalcules" (little animals); we now call them microorganisms, or microbes. Van Leeuwenhoek found them crawling everywhere—in pond water, rainwater, human sweat, and even in people's mouths. A new branch of science, microbiology, was born.

It was also the dawn of the industrial age, and cities were becoming overcrowded with people who didn't have access to proper sanitation. Child mortality soared and disease epidemics became more common. So society turned to microbiology to find the causes and cures of these threats. People wanted simple explanations and simple solutions.

Over the next two centuries, scientists would look to "germ theory" to explain infectious disease. In the 1860s, French biologist Louis Pasteur proved that puerperal fever, an illness to which women were susceptible to after giving birth, was caused by bacteria. This made it official: Microbes caused disease, and society was going to wage war on them.

There were undoubtedly a number of benefits that came from a greater understanding of bacteria's role in disease. Cities established better public sanitation and isolated their water supplies from sewage, which reduced the number of epidemics. Doctors disinfected their surgical instruments and operating theaters, which lowered the rate of hospital deaths. And Alexander Fleming's discovery of penicillin in 1928 led to antibiotics that reduced the number of deaths from diseases caused by microorganisms.[2] For a time, it looked like the war was all but won.

The sharp decline in the rate of deaths from infectious diseases reinforced the general belief that microbes were harmful in basically all cases. And for the most part, the 19th-century perception of bacteria as present only in the case of disease has persisted and is still with us today. This belief influences our lives in many meaningful ways. The pavement we walk on is treated with detergent. We fastidiously wash ourselves with antibacterial soaps and apply antibacterial lotions. We treat farm animals with antibiotics and rush to take antibiotics ourselves, even for viral infections.

The 1950s—A new understanding of microbes

In the 1950s, to learn more about microorganisms, scientists developed a way to raise lab animals in microbe-free environments. They delivered the animals in sterile conditions via cesarean section, weaned them on formula, then continued growing them in a completely sterile environment.[3]

Because they thought microorganisms were solely parasites, these scientists expected to raise extremely healthy, robust animals. To their unpleasant surprise, the animals proved extremely susceptible to disease; their immune systems were underdeveloped. Even more surprisingly, they had thin intestinal walls, their hearts pumped blood more slowly than normal, and they weighed noticeably less.

Suddenly it was apparent that microbes had been good for something after all.

The *Helicobacter* bacterium—Dr. Jekyll and Mr. Hyde?

Australians are known for their maverick outlook—think Crocodile Dundee and Steve Irwin—which doesn't exactly match the deliberate, empirical approach of science. But it took this Aussie mentality to finally correct one of the biggest misconceptions about the role of bacteria in the body.

For a long time, scientists thought that since the human stomach is full of acid, no life could survive inside it, including bacteria. Cue two Australian scientists, Barry Marshall and Robin Warren, who in 1982 discovered *Helicobacter pylori*, a spiral-shaped bacterium, in the stomachs of people who suffered from gastritis (inflammation of the stomach) and peptic ulcers (erosions in the stomach lining, which often cause pain and bleeding).

Since most people thought nothing could live inside the stomach, the scientific community ridiculed the assertion that *H. pylori* was related to the illnesses. But Marshall and Warren were determined to prove otherwise. Ever the reckless Aussies, they took it upon themselves to grow the bacteria in broth and then drink it. Of course, they both immediately became violently ill with gastritis. But when antimicrobial agents cured both of them and they reproduced their results in volunteers, it was established that *Helicobacter pylori* did in fact cause gastritis and gastric ulcers.

Marshall and Warren had proven something huge: Microbes were living inside our digestive system. In 2005, some 20 years after literally eating bacteria to prove their point—and after the scientific community had had enough time to digest their findings—the two Aussies won the Nobel Prize in Physiology or Medicine for their work.

We now know that more than 50 percent of all people have *H. pylori* in their upper gastrointestinal tract.[4] Somewhat ironically, we also know that while it *can* cause disease, more than 80 percent of people who have it in their gut never develop symptoms.[5]

It turns out that *H. pylori* isn't a single bacterium, but several species of bacteria that have lived in harmony in our stomachs for a very long time. In fact, *H. pylori* isn't really an "infectious" agent at all. It only becomes a problem when there's an imbalance of its different strains, when its harmful strains grow too much and cause a gastric disorder.

It's as if some strains of *H. pylori* are house cats and some are tigers. Theoretically, you can keep both species as pets, as long as you keep the tiger chained or caged. But if the tiger somehow breaks free and is left to its own devices, it can inflict some serious damage.

Infectious diseases do largely come from unwanted microbes that invade the population from outside. But for the most part, all of the microbes *inside* us are necessary for good health, and they even help protect us from harmful invaders. The catch is that the different strains inside our body have to maintain a delicate balance. When they're out of balance, a state called dysbiosis, they too can cause disease.

THE IMPORTANCE OF BIODIVERSITY IN THE MICROBIOME

Chances are, you know some people who are very competitive and some who aren't. But as a whole species, humans are *very* competitive. When we move into an ecosystem, we don't hesitate to establish ourselves at the top of the food chain. We quickly kill off the most threatening predators around so they won't bother us or our livestock. We leave grass-eating animals alone so we can hunt them later. We rarely appreciate that disrupting the balance of the ecosystem is bound to come back to haunt us in the long run.

Hunters killed the last wolf living in Yellowstone National Park in 1926, removing the top predator in that specific ecosystem. Over the next decades, the elk population ballooned and their overgrazing steadily reduced the park's vegetation. Even as the elk continued to prosper, the destruction of the ecosystem caused other populations of animals to thin. The elk overran the vegetation that lined the riverbanks of the park, destroying the soil embankments to the point where even the rivers ran dry. It was clear that by killing off the wolves, hunters had disturbed a very important and delicate balance in the ecosystem.

In 1996, the gray wolf was reintroduced to Yellowstone. Now, more than 20 years later, the elk population is under control, and without human help, species that haven't been seen in years, including the red fox and beaver, have returned to their old habitats.[6] But most amazingly, after the wolf's reintroduction, the vegetation on the riverbanks also grew back and the rivers started to flow naturally again, eventually recovering in full. Once the species of the ecosystem were back in balance, the environment was able to heal itself.

I think the story of the gray wolf in Yellowstone is a very strong parallel for the story of the human microbiome, the vast ecosystem of microbes living inside us. The universal rule of any ecosystem—whether it's a forest, a coral reef, or the microbes inside us—is that the more diverse it is, the more resilient it and its inhabitants are. Life on earth thrives when all the species in a system balance each other out.

Since we didn't know any better, we spent a great deal of our recent past killing off the bacteria that we thought were our body's most significant predators. But now we know that while certain bacteria *can* be a serious threat to our health, bacteria themselves are not such a black-and-white issue. They're a lot more like the gray wolf of Yellowstone, crucial for maintaining the balance of our microbiome and for protecting our overall health.

WHY OUR MOUTHS NEED BACTERIA

Nearly every dentist has wondered why a person who brushes more and eats less sugar can get decay and a person who brushes less and eats *more* sugar might not have any decay at all. (In 2016, the Food and Drug Administration or FDA went so far as to take flossing off its list of recommendations for preventing oral disease, simply because scientific research hasn't been able to conclusively prove that it actually decreases the chances of dental diseases like decay and gum disease.)[7] Early theories dismissed this paradox by attributing tooth decay to infection. It was known that the bacterium *Streptococcus mutans* caused decay.

But since then, research has revealed that many more species are involved and that the bacteria in the mouth *change* during the various disease states.[8]

When it comes to bacteria and tooth decay, it's more a matter of maintaining a *balance* among the different species than it is of fighting back invaders. (In reality, just as *H. pylori* lives in healthy stomachs, *S. mutans* lives in healthy mouths.) A lot of this balancing takes place in the plaque on our teeth. That's right—even plaque plays a role in our oral health.

Plaque is commonly described as "a sticky film." But it's actually a little more complicated than that. Plaque is built up by bacteria that release acids after you eat sugar, and it can keep these acids in contact with your teeth. Over time the acids can break down the enamel and cause cavities.

But thanks to our new understanding of the human microbiome, we now know that plaque also helps to maintain our teeth. In order to acknowledge that, we now refer to it as *dental biofilm*. (Biofilm is a layer of microbes that stick to a surface.)[9] The mouth is an extremely difficult place to live, what with our chewing, digestion, speaking, and breathing. To survive, microbes build little houses—biofilms—to protect themselves.

To beat tooth decay, we need to appreciate this delicate ecology of the mouth. Simply removing plaque, while useful, does not address the root cause of oral disease.

Bacteria manage the minerals in your teeth

Earlier I explained that the tooth has three main layers: the enamel, the dentin, and the pulp. The enamel is basically inanimate, while the dentin has cells called odontoblasts that protect both it and the pulp.

While the enamel doesn't have any live *human* cells in it, thousands and thousands of microbes are crawling up and down it at all times. These bacteria live on the surface of the tooth, building biofilm, and also within the hollow crystalline structure of enamel itself. And along with odontoblasts, they protect and maintain the enamel.

The enamel is in a constant state of flux, forever exchanging minerals and nutrients with your saliva. When you chew food, your salivary glands add enzymes to your saliva to start the process of digestion, which decreases the pH of the mouth. This shift in acidity can pull calcium and phosphorus out of the enamel and into our saliva.

When your mouth is healthy, bacteria help manage this exchange of minerals. In order to survive and to build their house of biofilm, they too need calcium. They share the calcium in our saliva with our teeth.

In order to prevent disease you need the microbes inside the mouth to stay in harmony. Your saliva gives them the minerals they need to build their house, and in a happy trade-off, the microbes help manage the supply chain of minerals that pass among your saliva, biofilm, and tooth enamel.

In our mouth and in the rest of our body, there are different types of bacteria. At a basic level, we can divide them into two groups—slow eaters and fast eaters. The fast eaters feed on simple carbohydrates like sugar. When we eat sugary and white flour–based foods, we send these bacteria into an eating frenzy. And when they metabolize sugars, they release acids.

These acids can act to pull calcium out of tooth enamel. But the microbes in the mouth all seem to know this; they provide a counterbalance by releasing calcium from saliva and their own biofilm reserves.[10] Overall, your teeth can handle a certain amount of sugar and the acids it helps produce.

But over time, if you eat too much sugar, the fast-metabolizing strains multiply too rapidly and spew out too much acid.[11] Eventually the bacteria run out of calcium from saliva and their biofilm reserves, and they're forced to start siphoning calcium from the only place left, the tooth enamel. If this process of acid release and calcium depletion continues for too long, bacteria eat away too much enamel, and bingo, you have tooth decay.

It's not simply that sugar combines with bacteria to create acid that decays the enamel. It's more that *too much* sugar sparks a chain reaction that leaches too much calcium from the enamel too quickly. Tooth decay isn't a bacterial infection. It's a condition where our diet has effectively forced the bacteria in our mouth into starvation. Our mouths simply weren't designed to deal with the imbalances created by the modern diet.

HOW THE INDUSTRIAL REVOLUTION CHANGED OUR MOUTH AND HEALTH

When did our diet stray from the foods that our mouths were designed to process? Researchers have studied the DNA of plaque that has survived on human skulls dating back to our distant ancestors. They've found that there were two major shifts in the diversity and composition of the oral microbiome in humans over the course of our time on earth—in other words, two major moments in human history where our diets went off course.[12]

The first shift came when humans stopped living as hunters and gatherers and started farming. Plaque from the skulls of people who lived as hunter-gatherers shows that they had much more diverse oral bacteria than their descendants who lived in agricultural societies. They also had far less decay, so it seems that as long as their oral microbiome was balanced and diverse, their dental (and probably digestive) health took care of itself. (I should note that the methods we have to measure bacteria in ancient plaque may have limitations. But studies have shown by other means as well that hunter-gatherers had more diverse microbiomes.)[13]

Scientists have analyzed the bacterium *Streptococcus mutans*, which plays a major role in tooth decay. They estimate that it expanded exponentially around 10,000 years ago. This would pin the start of modern dental disease, which is to say tooth decay, to roughly the same time period as the agricultural revolution, when the human diet significantly changed.

The second shift in our oral microbiome took place in the 1850s, during the Industrial Revolution. For the first time, people in the Western world had everyday access to white flour and refined sugar. Around the same time, the diversity of the bacteria in our oral microbiome decreased drastically.

White flour and refined sugar consist of simple carbohydrates that serve as instant fuel for certain kinds of bacteria, like *S. mutans* and *Lactobacillus acidophilus* (which, like *S. mutans*, participates in tooth decay). These bacteria grow at the expense of slower-growing microbes that are designed to digest longer, more complex molecules. The modernization of food disrupted the bacterial balance on a mass scale, and modern dental disease was born.

The thing that's important to remember, however, is that by themselves, simple carbs like sugar and flour don't cause as much damage to our teeth as most of us think. Rather, it's how they reduce the diversity of our oral microbiome that causes problems. And the same imbalance can happen in our gut, leading to more serious diseases.

Ancient dental disease: The exception that proves the rule?

While ancient populations were generally known to have little dental disease, exceptions have popped up in archaeological records. One population, which lived near the Grotte des Pigeons cave in Morocco around 13,000 to 15,000 years ago, had close to 100 percent tooth decay.[14]

Archaeologists looked at their dental plaque to extrapolate their diet and explain the anomaly. Generally, their diet appeared to contain a lot of legumes and wild oats. But it also contained a wild acorn, rich in sugar, that produced a sweet paste when it was cooked. This was the most likely cause of the decay.

This case is an outlier, but it helps show how modern access to sugars and carbohydrates might drive our own oral disease.

THE MOUTH-GUT AXIS—HOW ORAL BACTERIA DICTATE YOUR *BODY'S* HEALTH

Of course, bacteria play a role in managing more than our teeth. The oral microbiome flows beyond the mouth and into the digestive tract to become the gut microbiome. And it's there, deep in our digestive system, that microbes become profoundly important to the overall function of our body.

The simplest way to look at the human gut (digestive tract) is to imagine it as a tube-like conveyor belt that takes food from the mouth, processes it to create fuel, and then gets rid of the waste products through the opposite orifice. But the more we learn about the gut, the more we understand that, much like our skin, it's an organ that influences and contributes to crucial physiological processes throughout the body.

Instead of the more straightforward job of *protecting* us from the outside world, like a wall, our gut has to do a lot more nuanced work and a lot more multitasking. The gut has to transport, digest, and absorb nutrients while filtering out contaminants that shouldn't get into the bloodstream. On top of that, it has to signal to the rest of the body what's coming next.

The size of the gut should give you an idea of how big a job this all is. It has a surface area of approximately 32 meters squared,[15] and if you unfurled the digestive tract and laid it out flat, it would roughly cover half of a badminton court.

All of our organs and blood vessels and our entire gut are lined with epithelium cells. These cells act as a sort of gate that either allows outside molecules to pass through to the rest of the body or refuses them entrance. For an additional layer of protection and insulation, the gut is also lined with a layer of mucus that hydrates and nourishes the intestinal cells.

But as we've only recently discovered, the gut has something else to help it do its many jobs: a vast population of microflora— bacteria, viruses, fungi, and even more obscure organisms— that live in the gut lining. These living microorganisms serve as another protective barrier for our insides; they produce compounds that kill off potentially harmful bacteria, filter out damaging materials in food like heavy metals, and stimulate mucus production.

Your gut—as diverse as the Amazon and as populous as the Milky Way

Traditional societies generally had a better understanding of bacteria's role in a healthy diet than we do today, even if they didn't fully understand the ins and outs of it all.

Almost 2,500 years ago, Greek physician Hippocrates, considered the father of modern medicine, said, "All disease begins in the gut." In ancient medicine, the health of the digestive system was believed to be the key to overall well-being. (Note: When we say *gut*, we're referring to the whole gastrointestinal system: the stomach, small and large intestines, and the colon.)

Now we know that this ancient wisdom was on to something, as the digestive tract—or gut—houses the majority of the bacteria in our body. But in the two and a half millennia that followed the time of Hippocrates, as medical science advanced, gut health took a backseat to other areas of the body.

Today, scientists understand that as an ecosystem, the human gut is as diverse and complex as a lush tropical forest. The normal human microbiome—the population of microorganisms, or microbes, living inside us—consists of more than 1,000 species. They include bacteria, eukaryotes (cells with organelles and membranes), archaea (single-cell microbes that don't have a nucleus), viruses, and microscopic fungi.[16]

There are no fewer than 10^{11} to 10^{12} of cells per gram living in the colon.[17] That's close to the number of stars in the Milky Way. More than 70 percent of these microorganisms live in the colon, and bacteria make up 60 percent of all species in the gut. (Sixty percent of fecal matter is also bacteria.) These bacteria belong to at least 500 different species.

In 2008 the Human Microbiome Project set out to use genetic sequencing technology to map the human microbiome. So far it has been able to profile tens of thousands of microbial genes. Scientists believe that, in the end, the number of microbes we find living in our bodies will be staggering.

At the very least, microbes play a far greater role in our health than we ever realized.

Your mouth is the gatekeeper of your gut

The fact that your gut is filled with trillions of bacteria might be a little overwhelming. But what goes on in the gut is really just a continuation of what happens, on a smaller scale, in your mouth, where your microbiome starts. In fact, your microbiome *literally* started in your mouth.

In the womb, a child's digestive tract starts growing without microbes. The fetus receives nutrients from the placenta, and it depends on Mom to filter out any nasty bacteria from the environment.

But when a baby is born, it's thrown into a world that is crawling with bacteria. In fact, birth itself is designed to deliver a "starter" pack of microbes to a newborn child; the first microbes it encounters are those in the mother's vagina.[18]

The beginning of the child's life serves as a kind of crash course introduction to the world of microbes and how to deal with them. Breast-feeding plays a key role in this. Immune cells from a mother's gut can migrate to her mammary glands, and as a result, her breast milk will contain antibodies for certain microorganisms.[19]

The first place that these microbes colonize is, naturally, in the child's mouth. The oral microbiome then delivers certain bacteria to the gut microbiome. This "seeding" process means that in the first weeks to months of life, the mouth and gut microbiome are very similar. Eventually they become distinct systems, but their microbial populations always remain deeply connected.

This is how the trillions of microbes in your gut microbiome and immune system came about. The mouth acts as the first gateway to the gut microbiome, and it continues serving it throughout life. Every time you swallow saliva, you're sending thousands and thousands of bacteria to your gut.

No less than 80 percent of the body's immune cells live in the digestive system. The gut produces more antibodies than any other organ. When harmful microbes (whose molecules are similar but not identical to friendly gut microbes) try to invade the gut lining, our gut bacteria seem to help our immune system by sending messages that pass through the gut lining. These messages tell immune cells to bind to the harmful microbes, eat them, and dispose of them.[20]

But gut bacteria don't just influence immune cells in the gut. They can also send messages to immune cells in distant parts of the body. For instance, parts of the microbes' cell walls, which are made from an amino acid and sugar mesh called peptidoglycan, can activate immune cells located in bone marrow, in addition to other parts of the body.[21] Research has also shown that when bacteria in the gut consume fiber, they produce fatty acids that help manage the immune system and even metabolism.[22]

The body is in constant communication with the gut about what's coming into it from the outside world. And while the gut calls most of the plays, the playbook is largely written in the mouth. The healthier your mouth and oral microbiome, the healthier your gut, immune system, and entire body.

WHY FIBER IS IMPORTANT FOR A HEALTHY MOUTH AND GUT

The next time you sit down to a meal, remember that you're responsible for feeding trillions of tiny microbial lives with what's on your plate.

Generally speaking, your mouth contains "bad" bacteria that help cause tooth decay and "good" bacteria that not only manage calcium in your teeth but help to fight off the bugs that cause decay. The bad bacteria are fast metabolizers that feed on simple carbohydrates. The good (or "probiotic") bacteria are slower metabolizers that feed on complex carbohydrates, or fiber, turning it into short-chain fatty acids. (Certain probiotic gut bacteria perform this conversion via fermentation.)

If you don't eat enough fiber and instead eat mainly simple carbohydrates (sugar), you can cause the faster-metabolizing bacteria to grow and take over, causing more tooth decay. But the mouth is not the only place where the battle between good and bad bacteria—and between sugar and fiber—is waged. It also goes on in the gut.

We know that humans don't digest dietary fiber, but we've long known that it aids digestion. We've attributed that to the way it bulks up the stool, making it pass through the colon more easily. But it also feeds the good bacteria in the gut, which use it for energy and to maintain the all-important lining of the gut.[23]

Simple carbohydrates in the modern diet

Studies have shown that traditional diets high in natural sources of fiber—such as a variety of vegetables, nuts, seeds, and whole grains—gave our ancestors far more diverse gut bacteria than we have today.[24] Their balanced microbiomes meant that they didn't suffer from our rate of tooth decay, and were similarly unlikely to experience chronic digestive disorders like irritable bowel syndrome or ulcerative colitis.

But today, the average American adult eats only around 15 grams of fiber a day.[25] This amount pales in comparison with our distant ancestors, who ate around 100 grams per day.[26]

Again, we can trace this unfortunate shift in our diet to the Industrial Revolution and the modernization of food. In nature, sugar is usually locked up in plants, in a natural fiber casing. I like to think of this as "carbohydrates in context." It means that when people and animals consume plants in their natural form, their bodies can access their simple carbs only after first breaking down their fiber. This means the microbiomes in their mouth and gut naturally stay balanced.

But when industrialization gave us direct access to refined white sugar and flour, which supply the simple carbs without their natural plant casings, it threw our microbiomes out of balance. Our teeth, and the rest of us, suffered the consequences.

BLEEDING GUMS, YOUR GUT, AND YOUR IMMUNE SYSTEM

How bleeding gums can mean trouble in the gut

If your gums have ever bled when you brushed or flossed, you're familiar with inflammation. Simply put, tissue becomes inflamed when the body's immune cells flood it to fight off pathogens.

A certain amount of inflammation is normal. After all, your body is constantly interacting with foreign microbes. So when your gums bleed a little bit from brushing, it's usually not a sign of something serious. It just means that there's a bit of a microbial imbalance in your mouth, and a trip to the dentist and a bit more vigorous flossing and brushing will get it under control.

But gums that bleed *too much* are usually the first sign that your body is experiencing excess inflammation. If left untreated for enough time, bleeding gums can lead to periodontal (gum) disease. When you have gum disease, your gums are chronically inflamed and start to draw away from the teeth. Eventually the ligaments and jawbone that hold the teeth in place can weaken; in the worst-case scenario, the bone will be eaten away and the teeth will fall out. In the United States, 46 percent of adults suffer from some degree of gum disease, and 9 to 13 percent suffer from a severe form.[27]

Periodontal disease is extremely inconsistent and unpredictable. Like tooth decay, it spreads like wildfire in some people but can be managed with treatment, while in others it slowly progresses to an advanced state and basically refuses to respond to treatment.

The mouth is designed to exist in a state of low-grade inflammation, where the cells in the gums are forever reacting to the diverse mix of nutrients, minerals, enzymes, foreign bodies, and other substances that pass through.[28] But when this inflammation turns into gum disease, it's probably a sign that the mouth's microbiome is imbalanced and that your immune system is, in a sense, overreacting.

Since the gut is basically the control center for our immune system, periodontal disease is likely a sign that there's dysbiosis, an imbalance of good and bad bacteria, in the gut as well.

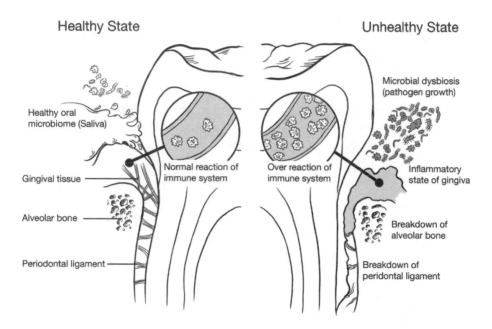

Fig. 15. Bleeding gums and your gut: how an imbalanced immune system drives gum disease

The bulk of the immune system lies in the gut and is separated from the gut microbiome by a one-cell-thick lining. The gut lining is like a fence over which your immune system and trillions of microbes communicate. The cells in the lining have to be bound together tightly for it all to work properly. This gut lining is meant to allow only small, selected molecules to cross the barrier at the junctions where the cells join one another and to keep everything else out.

But there are times when these epithelial cells are compromised and can't form an effective barrier. For example, the bacterium responsible for cholera, *Vibrio cholerae*, produces a toxin that causes the epithelial cells to leak ions inside the gut, resulting in diarrhea.[29]

Some medications, including aspirin and anti-inflammatory drugs like ibuprofen, can also make the gut barrier permeable. Excessive alcohol use can, too. These factors can lead to several unpleasant consequences, including local bowel inflammation and diarrhea. The good news is that stopping the cause of the irritation usually lets the gut heal and start working properly again.

The overuse of antibiotics, however, is another story. Antibiotics are like bacteria grenades, and too many of them can do long-term damage to the bacterial landscape of the gut, leading to more systemic, chronic problems.[30]

For example, antibiotics can disrupt bacteria that are supposed to "guard" the gut, leaving them unable to do their job. This in turn can cause the epithelial cells that form the gut lining to separate from one another and start dying, creating microscopic holes in the gut. A mix of semi-digested food and bacteria will then leak into the underlying tissue and into the blood vessels, hence the term "leaky gut."

Not consuming enough fiber can have a similar effect. If the good bacteria in your gut don't get enough fiber, they can shift into a kind of starvation mode in which they're forced to feed on mucin, a mucus-like coating that lubricates and protects the gut lining. If too much of that mucin is depleted, the gut barrier may not be able to function properly, resulting in digestive issues and leaky gut.[31]

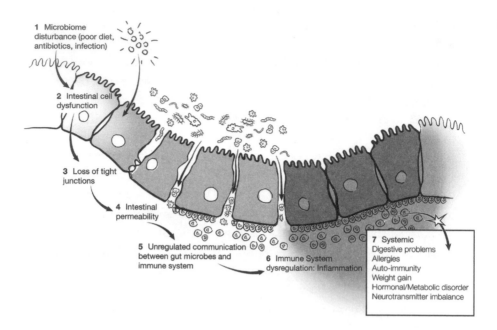

1 Microbiome disturbance (poor diet, antibiotics, infection)

2 Intestinal cell dysfunction

3 Loss of tight junctions

4 Intestinal permeability

5 Unregulated communication between gut microbes and immune system

6 Immune System dysregulation: Inflammation

7 Systemic
Digestive problems
Allergies
Auto-immunity
Weight gain
Hormonal/Metabolic disorder
Neurotransmitter imbalance

Fig. 16. Leaky gut: How intestinal permeability causes chronic disease

Leaky gut can disrupt the conversation between gut microbes and the immune system and trigger the immune system to over-react. The immune system can go haywire and spark allergic reactions,[32] weight gain,[33] and even mental disorders.[34] Bleeding gums can be among the first symptoms of the microbial imbalances that cause these conditions.

The gut and autoimmune disease

The mouth is one of our best measures of how well our immune system is working. When the immune system is healthy, immune cells target pathogens, like viruses. When there are no pathogens around, the immune cells lie in wait. But in an autoimmune disease, the immune cells stay active and attack healthy cells and proteins, which can lead to chronic inflammation and other problems.[35]

Autoimmune diseases have skyrocketed around the world since the end of World War II. More than 80 of these diseases have appeared since then, and conditions like Crohn's, rheumatoid arthritis, multiple sclerosis, and type I diabetes have become more and more common.[36,]

Since the gut and its microbes play such an important role in the regulation of the immune system, it stands to reason that the deterioration of the microbiome has contributed to this rise. In fact, recent studies have provided "clear and increasing evidence that changes in the microbiota are associated with . . . autoimmune diseases like type 1 diabetes, celiac disease, and rheumatoid arthritis."[37]

Our immune system relies on our gut microbes to relay information that helps it target pathogens and not our own cells. When that balance is off and the gut is leaky, immune cells start attacking healthy cells, and autoimmune diseases like the ones mentioned above can develop.

Early signs of autoimmune conditions often appear in the mouth. *Lichen planus*, an inflammatory condition of the skin and mucous membranes, provides a good example. In the mouth it turns up as a lacy or cotton-like white film on the inner cheek.[38]

Celiac disease, where the immune system attacks the digestive system when gluten is present, is another autoimmune disorder that often first shows itself in the mouth. It can often be identified in children who have malformed tooth enamel, mouth ulcers, or other oral lesions. The problem is that celiac disease often goes undiagnosed for many years, causing chronic illness.

Celiac disease is linked to other autoimmune disorders, like diabetes and thyroiditis. This suggests that celiac disease may share some common pathogenic gut imbalances with other autoimmune diseases.[39]

These microbial and immune system problems are also connected to chronic digestive diseases such as irritable bowel syndrome,[40] Crohn's disease,[41] and ulcerative colitis.[42]

I see many people who have battled chronic digestive conditions all their lives. The first symptoms of these conditions often arise in the mouth. But another thing they have in common is that they can all be prevented by feeding oral and gut bacteria the right way.

Gum disease and other chronic diseases

Every time you swallow, thousands of bacteria are sent through your digestive tract.[43] So when the microbiome in your mouth is out of balance, as it is when you have gum disease, the effects are felt all over your body.

For many years, research illuminated correlations between periodontitis and cardiovascular disease, rheumatoid arthritis, Alzheimer's disease, pulmonary disease, preterm delivery of low-birth-weight infants, and metabolic disease.[44] The exact mechanisms, however, are not yet fully understood.

When we look at gum disease through the lens of the microbiome, we see how microbial dysbiosis connects the dots between the mouth and illnesses throughout the body. The oral and gut microbiome are two distinct yet related species. We know that the oral microbiome acts to seed the empty gut microbiome in a newborn child. But this communication never really stops—it continues throughout your life.

Studies are now showing dysbiosis to the gut microbiome is linked to conditions like allergies,[45] type 2 diabetes,[46] obesity,[47] and even disorders of the brain[48] like ADHD, Alzheimer's disease, and dementia. The importance of the microbiome just can't be understated.

Your mouth serves as the bodyguard for your gut and the rest of your body for your entire life.

REPLENISHING YOUR MICROBIOME: FERMENTED FOOD

It's no coincidence that fermented foods used to be consumed across the globe in all civilizations.

Before the invention of refrigeration, fermentation was one of the few ways that people could make food last longer. Fermentation involves introducing beneficial bacteria to food in order to effectively cancel out the harmful microbes that cause food to spoil. So fermented foods are chock-full of probiotic bacteria and prebiotic fiber that help feed and balance the microbial colonies inside us.

The key lies within the chemistry of the many species of lactobacillus bacteria. Lactobacillus readily uses lactose or other sugars and converts it to lactic acid.[49] Lactic acid is a natural preservative that inhibits the growth of harmful bacteria. It also increases or preserves the enzymes and vitamins that aid digestion. When fresh vegetables weren't readily available throughout the year, traditional cultures often preserved them through fermentation.

Today, since we widely perceive bacteria as harmful, we've largely forgotten the art of fermenting foods and lost the bacterial diversity that comes with eating them. Due to improved transportation and storage, vegetables are now available year round, and we now preserve most of them through refrigeration and canning. Our dairy is boiled and homogenized, and our plants are sprayed with fertilizers.

These processes are great for the shelf life of foods and make them safer to transport, but they don't maintain a lot of the bacteria that's produced through fermentation—the bacteria our mouths and guts need to stay healthy.

HOW TO KEEP YOUR MICROBIOME BALANCED

In *The Dental Diet*, we'll focus on influencing your body's microbiota by consuming fiber, probiotics, and prebiotics. But the reality is that everything you do interacts with microbes. If you've had tooth decay in your life, it's in no small part due to a loss of bacterial diversity in your mouth. Research is revealing that there are some interesting nondietary ways that your lifestyle can create a diverse and strong microbiome.

Intermittent fasting

We know that our gut flora play an integral role in digestion, but this role extends to managing the entire metabolism of the body. When you eat, your flora have to work to break down and digest food, so your eating cycle will impact the day-to-day life of your microbiome.

Studies on mice have shown that time without food (fasting) increases bacterial diversity, suggesting that during the absence of food, bacteria keep working. In fact, the time without food represents a more natural feeding cycle (when food is not available) and allows microbes to do their own "spring cleaning" of our digestive and immune system, which is likely a part of our body's normal interaction with microflora.[50]

Stress

Having lots of different types of microbes helps our body stay resilient to outside stresses. Stress is something we were designed to encounter only rarely. Only rarely is our system meant to activate its fight-or-flight response.[51]

But today we have changed our exposure to stress. We're now exposed to constant, low-grade stress that is sending survival signals throughout our body. These signals seem to impact our microbiome as well. Animal studies have shown that a high-stress environment reduces bacterial diversity.[52] If you're constantly worrying about school, work, or your relationships, your microbiome is likely feeling the effects.

Sleep

Your digestive system works on a diurnal or circadian rhythm connected to the day–night cycle and sleep. When your sleep cycle is interrupted (you don't get enough or you get poor quality) your gut microbes suffer as a result.

Interestingly, new research is showing how gut microbes may even be in control of your diurnal rhythm. However, lack of sleep seems to change its diversity.[53]

Exercise

As if bacteria aren't doing enough already, they also may be checking that you're going to the gym. Like your other habits, how you move and condition your body via exercise may influence your microbiome. While your exercise performance may be influenced by how healthy your bacteria are, the relationship is likely a back-and-forth, with exercise providing a positive boost to beneficial strains and metabolites in the gut.[54]

Exposure to dirt

Yes, you read that right: getting dirty may be a crucial piece of your microbiome puzzle. Soil, or dirt, is formed by the interactions among microorganisms, minerals, dead plants, and animals. It supports life all over the earth. When we remove our exposure to soil, we may be removing a crucial boost to our own microbes. Soil and humans share species of microbes that are likely transferred when we eat an animal or plant.[55]

Getting your food from natural, organic sources and also having your own garden (where you touch the soil) may provide a healthy (if dirty) boost to your microbiome.

Social environment and pets

You share microbes with your partner as well as the people you come in close contact with on a regular basis: co-workers, people at the gym, even your pets. In fact, people who own dogs have been shown to have significantly more diverse skin microbiomes.[56]

◆ ◆ ◆

A MICROBIOME PERSPECTIVE ON HEALTH

The idea that we simply need to brush and floss to remove "harmful" tooth plaque is based on an outdated model of dental disease. Tooth decay and gum disease have long been understood to be caused by bacteria. But new advances in our understanding of the human microbiome show us that microbes play integral roles in the body. And while outside infections don't account for how noninfectious diseases arise, a lack of balance in our microbiome does.

It's as if our body is the host of a super-organ—a veritable rain forest of trillions of microbes inside us—that we are only beginning to understand. The mouth and gut form the housing for these tiny inhabitants, and their health reflects how our bodies' relationship with them is working.

Disease in the mouth is caused by an imbalance of microbes that also live and need to stay balanced in the gut. We can look at the microbial health of our mouth as a window into the microbial health of our gut and the overall state of our entire body.

When we get our mouth healthy, the rest of the body will follow. Food, which has the power to balance our oral and gut microbiomes, is our mouth's best medicine.

CHAPTER 6

IT'S NOT GENETIC

How Crooked Teeth
Are Caused by Poor Nutrition

As a dentist, I am quite sad when people tell me they feel that their oral health is "hopeless." When someone feels hopeless about their health, it often turns into a vicious cycle of sadness and sickness. They think that because of their genetics, they'll have problems with their teeth no matter what, so they don't take proper care of them. Then they suffer from decay and other issues, which confirms their negative feelings. The whole thing is a self-fulfilling prophecy.

I have to admit that for a long time, I felt that some patients were predisposed to have oral health problems. My training had taught me as much. It seems like we've all concluded, at one time or another, that when it comes to dental health, genetics is destiny. Maybe good food, exercise, and healthy living can help you improve your health a little bit here and there, but it all amounts to nibbling around the edges. DNA is fate, and there's no changing fate.

When I first explain to people that if they eat certain foods they can truly improve the health and structure of their mouth, they're usually surprised.

It's true that DNA is a huge factor in how our bodies develop and in the overall state of our health. But while many people think it's like a computer code that gives our bodies directions they can't stray from, it's actually more like a blueprint that our bodies *interpret*. One of the best ways to make sure that our bodies interpret those directions in a healthy way is to give them the right nutrients.

While this may sound like a new idea, like many of the concepts we've talked about, there's been evidence for this for quite some time. One particular case involved a scientist called Francis Pottenger and a whole heap of cats. Today he might have been labeled a crazy cat person. But I'll let you be the judge.

POTTENGER'S CATS

In the 1930s, Dr. Pottenger carried out a 10-year, multiple-generation experiment on cats that showed, in very stark relief, how diet can affect biology.

Pottenger did experiments on cats that called for removing their adrenal glands. He fed them milk and cooked meat scraps as they recovered from surgery. But eventually he ran out of the cooked meat, so he ordered raw meat from a local supplier and fed it to some of the cats. To Pottenger's surprise, the cats that were fed the raw meat recovered from the surgery much faster than the others.[1]

Pottenger then began doing controlled experiments with cats and different foods. Over 10 years he studied the effects of raw and cooked meat as well as raw (unpasteurized), processed, and condensed milk on some 900 cats. The results were nothing short of stunning.

The cats that fed mostly on raw milk and meat remained relatively strong and healthy over generations. But the cats that consumed mostly cooked meats and processed and condensed milk had offspring that suffered from significant health problems.

The first generation developed crooked teeth and inflamed gums. The next generation weighed, on average, 20 percent less at birth and had severe skeletal problems. Their skulls, including their cheekbones and sinuses, were deformed, thin, and weak. It turned out that they had less calcium in their bones than normal cats did.

The third generation was even worse off. And the fourth generation of cats fed on cooked meat and pasteurized milk died out before any one of them reached six months of age.

Pottenger demonstrated how the wrong food can have a swift and devastating impact on a cat's health. That made him wonder if the right food could have a *positive* impact. To answer that question, he took some of the third generation of sickly cats and put them on the diet of raw dairy and meat. He also gave the generations that followed them that diet.

Sure enough, each new generation turned out healthier than the one that came before it. In the end, it took four generations feeding on the raw diet to bring the line back to normal health.

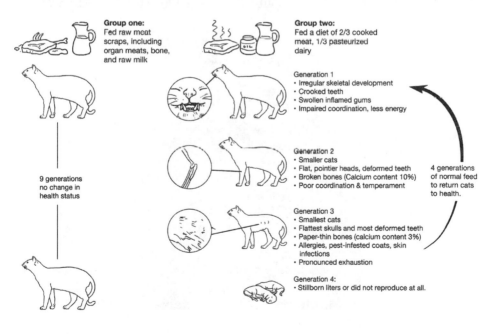

Fig. 17. Pottenger's cats: A 10-year study into the epigenetic impact of food

HOW YOUR ENVIRONMENT INFLUENCES YOUR HEALTH

As mentioned, DNA is more like a blueprint our bodies interpret than a commandment stating our unchangeable destiny. The study of how that interpretation works is called epigenetics. (The word comes from Greek, roughly translating to "above/on top of/ in addition to genetics." The more we learn about it, the more it seems that the way we live and how we eat can certainly change the way our DNA is expressed.

Pottenger himself had no way of knowing it, but his experiment was a strong testament to the power of epigenetics. The cats' DNA hadn't changed across the four generations, but the way in which their DNA was *expressed* changed for the worse, simply because he had fed them food that their bodies weren't designed for.

Why don't our bodies build bones like they used to?

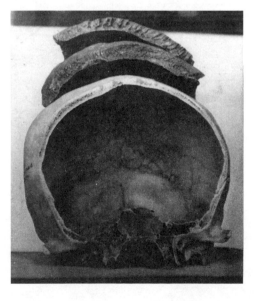

Fig. 18. Not just in cats: A comparison of the thickness of modern skulls and ancestral skulls by Weston A. Price

Years ago I saw a patient named Brian. Brian was referred to me for wisdom tooth removal by another dentist in my practice.

When Brian walked in, my heart rate went up. Yes, Brian was a big man. He was a huge, lumberjack-like figure. But the thing that unnerved me was that his head was *enormous*! Brian's head was as big and round as a bowling ball. Brian had grown up on his parents' farm and lived purely on foods they grew and raised themselves.

Brian wanted one of his wisdom teeth taken out because it needed a root canal. He preferred to have the tooth out than go through the procedure.

I was struck that all of Brian's wisdom teeth were fully erupted. Today I don't see a lot of jaws that are big enough to fully accommodate all four wisdom teeth. The bone surrounding Brian's bad tooth was thick and plentiful. I also found that his jaw was so big, my instruments could barely reach that tooth!

Today when I remove wisdom teeth from young adults, I see that the bone is thin and their jaws are tiny. It occurred to me that Brian's upbringing had provided him with the foods that gave his bones and teeth the minerals they needed to be strong and healthy.

THE EPIGENETICS OF CROOKED TEETH

Dr. Dave Singh was one of the early innovators in the field of craniofacial and epigenetic orthodontics. At his facilities in Beaverton, Oregon, he trains dentists in epigenetic orthodontics, showing them how we can take advantage of epigenetics to remodel our jaw and airways. He believes epigenetics is the most logical explanation for malocclusion. Yet today, even though roughly three-quarters of kids today develop crooked teeth, dental textbooks focus on classifying the *degree* of malocclusion rather than explaining how it comes about in the first place.

Dr. Singh believes malocclusion is a perfect example of our body using epigenetics to adjust to the environment. He defines the epigenetics of crooked teeth as "a solution for a complex system to remain in homeostasis, even when some of its components are imbalanced." He explains by using a construction analogy.

"When you're building a house, you start by building the foundations, then the walls, then the roof, and so on. The last thing you work on is the interior, which, in our body's case, includes the teeth. Our body can't *start* with the teeth and make sure they're straight, because then it might not have enough material to build the foundation that would match them. It might throw the whole house off. So the body starts with the jaw, it builds that as best it can with the resources it has, and at the end it installs the teeth. If the jaw ends up misshapen, the only way the teeth can go in is crooked, and that's how they go in."

The mouth appears to be the first place where we can evaluate the epigenetic messages that our cells and DNA are receiving from our food. It's the proverbial canary in the coal mine of our health.

After the Industrial Revolution, when we collectively switched from whole foods to processed foods, our jaws stopped developing as they had for thousands of years. Since then, as our diets have become even more unnatural, our modern epidemic of dental disease has only gotten worse. The deterioration is eerily reminiscent of Pottenger's cats. When we break down the general diet that most people in the West subsist on today, it's no wonder that our children have crooked teeth and tiny jaws.

DNA AND EPIGENETICS

How DNA works

Your body is made up of billions of cells. Each cell plays a little part in something your body does—everything from transporting oxygen to fighting infection, from storing a memory to building a tooth. Your body is an infinitely complex construction project that's constantly in flux, and your cells are the workers making everything happen.

But unlike a construction site, your body doesn't have a foreman or architect directing the cells, or workers, what to do. Instead, each cell follows the blueprint that's inside it, better known as DNA.

Each piece of your DNA is made of a very thin thread that's coiled up in the nucleus, or center, of the cell. The simplest way to describe the function of DNA is to say that it has a code printed on it. The code is actually made out of just four "letters," which represent four molecules used again and again in different combinations, millions and millions of times over. Sections of the code that spell a complete "word"—or, more accurately, an instruction—are called genes.

Genes tell your cells—your body's tiny workers—what to do. Again, that's everything from helping to clot your blood when you get cut to contracting your leg muscles when you run or determining the color of your eyes. Essentially, your cells do all of these different things by teaming up with other cells and producing different proteins, which, to put it very simply, serve as the raw materials and tools of the construction project that's you. Every cell in your body has the same set of genes; the reason your toe cells are different from tooth cells is that they use different genes to produce different proteins.

What's amazing is that the DNA of all living organisms— from a tiny paramecia to a palm tree to a pelican to you and me—uses the same four letters for its genetic code. In each organism, these simply spell out different instructions (genes). In a house cat, those genes instruct their cells to make a house cat. In a cheetah, they order up a cheetah. In us, they give instructions for making a person. We call the complete code of DNA inside us the human genome.

When American biologist James Watson and English physicist Francis Crick discovered the structure of DNA, in 1953—and therein the potential to decode it—medical science was launched into a DNA model of medicine. Much as we had begun to look for a microbe to explain every disease, we looked for a gene to explain every human characteristic.

In 1990 geneticists started working on the Human Genome Project, an international effort to decipher the entire sequence of human DNA, identifying each individual gene (instruction) and determining what each gene is responsible for. As different people, we all have different genomes, so the purpose of mapping the entire code is to discover every separate gene and figure out every different possible combination.[2]

Geneticists were extremely confident about the potential of the Human Genome Project. It was amazing, the idea that we could understand the code of life like we understand the code of a computer. As Stephen L. Talbott wrote of geneticists in *The New Atlantis*: "[T]hey heralded one revolutionary gene discovery after another—a gene for cystic fibrosis . . . a gene for cancer, a gene for obesity, a gene for depression, a gene for alcoholism, a gene for sexual preference. Building block by building block, genetics was going to show how a living organism could be constructed from mindless, indifferent matter."[3]

In 1992, Nobel Prize–winning geneticist Walter Gilbert wrote that he would one day be able to hold in his hand a CD with the human DNA sequence stored on it and announce: "Here is a human being; it's me!"[4]

Geneticists expected to find around 100,000 genes in the human genome, with some estimates going as high as two million. They reasoned that it would take that many genes to detail the construction of a species as diverse and complex as human beings. But when the Human Genome Project was finally completed in 2004, it looked like there must have been some kind of mistake. It turned out that we humans have only around 20,000 to 25,000 different genes in our DNA. That's around the same number as mice have.[5]

In reality, our cells don't use specific genes to create the traits, organs, and other characteristics that make us unique. It appears that they use *combinations* of specific genes, and the environment influences those combinations much more than we thought. In the age-old debate of nature versus nurture, we now understand that nurture has the stronger say in genetic expression.

To continue with our construction analogy, there is a set of genes that instruct your bone-making cells to build a jawbone, but how they carry out that task—how they set the dimensions of the jawbone—depends on the resources they're provided, the environmental conditions, and the feedback coming from their supervisor. The final outcome of the project is called gene expression.

How epigenetics works

If DNA isn't giving our cells specific instructions for each task they carry out, how *do* they know what to do?

Remember that I said the DNA is coiled up in the nucleus of the cell? The cell's organelles, the organs of the cell that do its work, need to read that blueprint to know what to do. How do they read the messages? The answer is another molecule called ribonucleic acid, or RNA. RNA makes copies of the DNA instructions and carries them to the organelles.

Up until a few years ago, we assumed that DNA wasn't just the blueprint but also the contractor. We thought that DNA basically "chose" the instructions it gave to the RNA to send to the rest of the cell.

Here's where it gets a little tricky: DNA doesn't choose which parts of itself get copied by RNA, and RNA doesn't, either. In reality, these choices are mostly the result of chemical reactions that begin outside the cell itself, are interpreted and relayed by the cell membrane, and then flow to the nucleus, where the DNA is stored.[6]

The outside of the cell (membrane) is equipped with hundreds of thousands of receptor proteins that are responsible for receiving different signals, like those delivered by nutrients, hormones, or neurotransmitters.[7] When an outside signal binds to these receptor proteins, they send a cascade of chemicals to the nucleus. This is the first whisper in a complex game of telephone that more or less determines which parts of the DNA end up being copied by the RNA and which parts of the RNA are used by the organelles to blurt out a new protein.

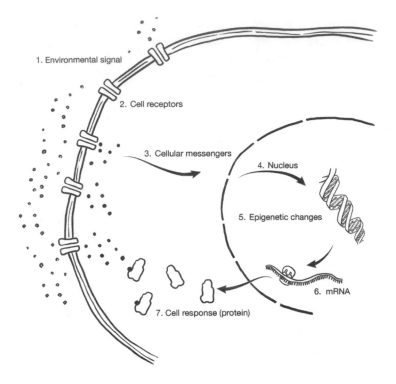

1. Environmental signal

2. Cell receptors

3. Cellular messengers

4. Nucleus

5. Epigenetic changes

6. mRNA

7. Cell response (protein)

Fig. 19. How the environment changes the DNA in your cells

Your environment literally changes how your genes are expressed. And your environment includes, crucially, the foods you choose to eat.

THE DUTCH HUNGER FAMINE

Pottenger gave us a fairly straightforward example of epigenetics at work—in cats. But we also have an example of how epigenetics can affect humans. It came in the form of the Dutch Hunger Winter, which took place in the Netherlands in 1944 to 1945.[8]

At that time, during the last years of World War II, the western part of the country was still occupied by Germany. A blockade cut off food supplies to the region, and people had access to only about 30 percent of the food they usually had. Eventually the entire population was at the brink of starvation, and people were forced to forage for any food they could find, even eating things like grass and tulip bulbs. Before the Allies liberated the region and restored the food supply in May 1945, around 20,000 people died.

Epidemiologists, who study how diseases originate and evolve, have used health records to study the long-term effects of the famine on the Dutch people.

One thing they observed is that babies who were conceived before or around the beginning of the famine and whose mothers were malnourished for the last few months of pregnancy were born abnormally small. On the other hand, babies who were conceived toward the end of the famine and whose mothers were malnourished for only the first few months of pregnancy were born with normal-size bodies.

It seems that the babies who were malnourished at the beginning of their gestation were able to "catch up" to normal birthweight, while the babies who were malnourished toward the end could not. That's intuitive enough. But as both sets of babies grew into adults, the effects of the famine seemed to stay with them throughout their entire lives.

The underweight babies stayed relatively small for the rest of their lives, even though they had access to a normal amount of food for all of that time. Meanwhile, the babies who were born at normal weights, having "caught up" in utero after being malnourished for the first few months of gestation, had higher obesity rates in adulthood. They suffered from other chronic health issues at higher rates as well. Why did that happen?

The answer appears to be a form of epigenetics called methylation. Methylation is like a set of chemical tags that attach to DNA. Each DNA molecule has many, many tags attached to it, and they influence how that DNA is expressed. Different combinations of tags produce different effects.

Researchers who studied survivors of the Dutch Hunger Famine found the children exposed to famine in the first trimester had less DNA methylation on the gene known to influence their insulin growth factor hormone.[9] That hormone determines whether the body uses glucose (sugar) for energy or stores it as fat. The methylation explains why one group was potentially more prone to putting on weight than the other over the long term.

Notably, Audrey Hepburn was a child of the Dutch Hunger Famine. It's eerie to think that the delicate facial features she was so famous for might have been a product of the epigenetic duress she and her mother experienced due to starvation. Hepburn suffered from health problems for most of her life; it's possible that while her body used nutrients efficiently, keeping her lean and delicate, it overcompensated in other ways, leading to complications. She died from a rare form of abdominal cancer in 1993.

THE GRANDMOTHER EFFECT—WHY YOUR GRANDMOTHER'S LIFE IMPACTS YOURS

We now know that epigenetic markers, or "edits," can be inherited by children, grandchildren, and the generations that come after them. But they can also be corrected. Studies have shown, for instance, how epigenetics shaped by smoking can be inherited and cause asthma:[10]

- If your grandmother was a smoker but your mom wasn't, you're 1.8 times more likely than average to suffer from asthma.
- If your mom smoked while she was pregnant with you, you're 1.5 times more likely than average to suffer from it.
- If both your grandmother and your mom smoked, you're 2.6 times more likely than average to develop the respiratory disease.

This all makes sense when you think about it. If Grandma was a smoker, her epigenetics likely "thought" she lived in a low-oxygen environment. They would have directed the cells that created and maintained her lung and airway tissues to adjust accordingly. Those adjustments would be passed down to your mother, but since your mother's cells would receive them while they were still very young and impressionable, their effects would seem to be heightened in her. And the same would be true for you, the grandchild.

Asthma is, after all, an inflammation of the tissue of the airways. In other words, it's an overreaction in that tissue to the *environment*.

COUNTLESS COMBINATIONS

The more we explore how epigenetics works, the more we see how complicated it really is. Epigenetics is a constant interaction of our genes with the environment. It impacts our health across the entire human life span—from our parents' lives leading up to conception, to the womb and birth, then childhood and adolescence, and throughout our adult lives.[11]

The food we eat has a large influence on our epigenetics. Natural food that has not been processed or refined contains nutrients that bring out the best in our epigenetic messaging. But altered food, such as much of the mass-produced food so many of us eat today, contains compounds that, almost like a computer virus, interfere with healthy epigenetic messaging.

HOW EATING AND BREATHING
CAN STRAIGHTEN YOUR TEETH

Dentists see all kinds of crooked teeth. There are jaws without sufficient space for upper teeth, and there are jaws without enough space for lower teeth. There are upper and lower jaws where the teeth just don't fit together. There are jaws so small that many of the teeth are completely buried in the gums.

Our skeletal system is remarkably intelligent and reactive. It unquestionably adjusts to our environment. Issues in our jaws and skulls are remarkable examples of how, when we don't eat the right food, our body responds accordingly.

As we're learning, the epigenome of our jaws, teeth, and airways is influenced by numerous environmental factors. These include many of the processes and hard substances we've discussed in previous chapters, including:

- *Breathing*—Nasal breathing lets our body use more oxygen and provides physical feedback, which influences our epigenetics.

- *Chewing*—Chewing whole, natural food provides exercise to our muscles for epigenetic feedback.

- *Vitamin D*—Helps the body absorb calcium, the building block of the skeletal system, and activates thousands of genes that influence the body right down to cell growth and differentiation.

- *Vitamin A*—Supports bone development through cell turnover and with vitamin D activates growth and development genes throughout the body.

- *Vitamin K2*—Is the bone development support factor for vitamins D and A that activates the proteins to direct calcium to the right places.

- *The microbiome*—The microbes inside us receive epigenetic messages from the food we eat and pass them on to our own genes.

EPIGENETICS AND CHRONIC DISEASE

Epigenetics doesn't just show how our teeth have degenerated. It shows how our entire body has changed. A host of new studies are demonstrating how epigenetic signals can increase our risk of suffering from chronic diseases:

- DNA methylation can trigger specific immune cells called T-lymphocytes to attack healthy cells, leading to autoimmune disorders.[12]

- DNA Methylation and histone modification (the molecules that the DNA is wrapped around) have been linked to insulin resistance and diabetes.[13]

- The misregulation of epigenetic mechanisms has been linked to cancer.[14]

- People who suffer from obesity and diabetes show distinct epigenetic marks. And there's evidence that the epigenetic processes linked to these diseases are influenced by environmental factors and diet.[15]

Epigenetics is teaching us that, just as our diet can help us strengthen our jaws and teeth, it can also help us fight chronic illnesses. It's showing us that we do have the power to change the genetic cards we were dealt—or at least how our body plays them. The answer isn't to find the newest medication to dull the symptoms. Instead, we need to appreciate that food shapes our health throughout our life by speaking directly to our genes.

A good way to understand epigenetics

A good way to understand epigenetics is to picture billions of little on–off switches inside your body that control everything from your stress response to how your body makes energy from food to your brain chemistry to how your liver detoxifies your system.

Now let's say a section of your DNA spells the word *printable*.

Two epigenetic processes—methylation (where the DNA is "edited" by a chemical reaction) and histone modification (a reaction that changes which parts of the DNA are exposed for RNA to copy)—can turn "letters" in the code on or off so it displays recognizable words like:

- Printable
- Print
- Table
- Tab
- Able

But methylation and histone modification could also edit the *printable* code so it creates unrecognizable words, like:

- Rin
- Tabl
- Ble
- Pri
- Inta

This is one reason why a single gene can lead to the creation of many, many different versions of the same protein—some healthy, some harmful—and it helps explain why the Human Genome Project found such an unexpectedly small number of human genes.

THE EPIGENETIC LANGUAGE OF FOOD

Every living organism contains epigenetic messages. These messages are passed down to it by its ancestors and introduced by the other organisms it eats for food and by its environment. And we humans are no exception.

When you eat an animal or vegetable, your body is listening to the epigenetic messages of its life, which are shaped by where it was raised and how it lived. Your body uses this information for its own health. This is one of the many reasons why the food you eat is so important.

Food sourcing for healthy epigenetics

The epigenetic influence of food cannot be understated.

Take fresh garlic, for instance. If we put it in hot oil or hot foods right away, we destroy its ability to produce allicin, an important cancer-fighting compound. But if you simply chop it and set it aside for 10 minutes, during the time that it's resting, the garlic makes copious amounts of allicin. And once it forms, it is not destroyed by later cooking.[16]

There are many ways you can influence the epigenetic influence of your food:

1. **Eat food that's organically grown with natural farming practices.**

   Plant foods should come from natural soil that contains a natural microbiome, without pesticides and other chemicals, nourished by insects, sunlight, fresh air, and CO_2. Naturally grown plants will pass along healthy epigenetic messages and nutrients to animals that eat them.

   You may see the largest, most perfectly shaped fruits and vegetables in the supermarket. But the reality is that this is not how nature prepares them, and the epigenetic messages they contain are not as compatible with our bodies as produce grown naturally.

   In nature, tomatoes are the size of cherries, or even smaller. In fact, small varieties of tomatoes are more nutritious than larger varieties. Lycopene is the most important phytonutrient in tomatoes, and a small cherry tomato might have 20 times more lycopene than a large supermarket tomato that was created by human agriculture.[17]

   Similarly, an animal that's raised on natural plants will have healthier epigenetics itself. So it's important to eat organic meats from animals that fed on plants in natural environments (like pasture-raised chickens, cows, and pigs).

2. **Eat locally sourced food.**

   The average vegetable on our supermarket shelves today has anywhere from 5 percent to 40 percent less mineral content than those of 50 years ago.[18] One reason for this is how far it usually travels before it gets to the supermarket, or how it's stored.

   Plants can lose 30 percent of their nutrients just three days after harvest.[19] Vegetables can lose 15 to 55 percent of their vitamin C, for instance, within a week. Some spinach can lose 90 percent of vitamin C within the first 24 hours after harvest. So if they have to be shipped a long way, or if they're stored in a refrigerator for a long time before they're put on the shelf or eaten, vegetables can become nutritional shells of what they were when they were picked.

3. **Eat seasonally.**

    All plants go through a similar life cycle: sprouting, leafing, flowering, fruiting, and then stockpiling sugars in their roots. Leafy greens grow in the spring. Broccoli and tomatoes are best in summer. Pumpkin and other root vegetables contain large amounts of stored nutrients for fall and winter.

    You should avoid food that sits on supermarket shelves or comes from factories that treat it with synthetic pesticides and antibiotics to keep it edible year-round.

EPIGENETICS—A NEW HOPE

Epigenetics is helping scientists fill in the gaps in our understanding of how the environment and the foods we eat influence our health. Crooked teeth are an illustration of epigenetics' power. Our body uses the information and resources it receives and makes the most workable solution for a given situation.

Tooth decay also provides a vivid picture of the interaction between our body and environment. But if you are healthy, with the right epigenetic inputs, cavities should never happen. Our teeth, and the immune cells that protect them, make up living systems that depend on fat-soluble vitamins to use minerals effectively and fight off potential invaders. At the same time, our mouth is an ecosystem of bacteria that actually live in harmony with our teeth, helping to put calcium where it's needed and to balance out the bad guys.

Our body and our microbiome talk to each other through the language of epigenetics, and they themselves are built, shaped, and maintained by genes that communicate through the language of epigenetics.

It's the most complex game of telephone ever played, and the food we eat carries nutrients that go a long way toward shaping those messages.

PART II

HOW MODERN FOOD HAS DESTROYED OUR HEALTH

CHAPTER 7

WHY THE FOOD ON YOUR PLATE IS MAKING YOU SICK

When I see patients who have lived with dental disease all their lives, we discuss their diet. They're always aware their diet is a problem—even if they haven't associated it with the poor condition of their mouth. They've usually tried diets that didn't work, or they feel paralyzed by all the information out there. Either way, they don't end up changing what they eat very much, if they change anything at all.

I feel for them, because it's not entirely their fault. Modern society has created this trap. We are now surrounded by food that barely resembles what humans ate for thousands of years. Today eating unhealthy food is harder to avoid than getting tooth decay, needing braces, or having your wisdom teeth pulled.

It's remarkable how little research, if any at all, has been done on the connection between our unnatural diets and our declining dental health. And while there's plenty of dietary and nutritional information out there telling people that eating processed, refined, or otherwise manipulated food is unhealthy, there's much less information on how to *break* these bad habits. (If you've ever been frustrated by this state of affairs, read on. The Dental Diet will help you sort it all out.)

We're effectively a species that has forgotten how to feed itself. Food may be easier to attain than ever, but our understanding of food seems to be at an all-time low. We're not able to make the simple changes to our habits that would help us escape the cycle of disease because, as a general population, we don't have a clear understanding of what actions we need to take.

The first step to solving any problem is to acknowledge there's an issue in the first place. In order to refrain from harming our body through food and to begin making every meal a boost to our genetic health, we need to understand the difference between our diet today and what made us healthy for thousands of years.

WHY TODAY'S "FOOD" ISN'T FOOD

There's something powerful about sitting around a table with other people over food. We have felt the power of food since we began walking the earth. And over thousands of years, the different cultures and societies of the world have carefully cultivated their relationship with food. Cultures have placed as much importance on passing food wisdom from generation to generation as they have religious customs and scientific knowledge. For most of our time on earth, food was treated as nothing less than sacred.

Our forebears had two very good reasons to treat it that way. The first was that, until the Industrial Revolution, food was a precious commodity. Imagine how special you'd think food was if you couldn't get it at the local supermarket and had to hunt or farm for it.

The second reason was that our ancestors couldn't afford to ignore, or consider only casually, the sourcing and preparation of their food. Without the luxury of modern science and medicine, they knew that their health, and that of their children, depended mainly on what they ate. That made them incredibly connected to the way food exists in nature, as our bodies are meant to process it.

The Industrial Revolution changed all that. No longer did food need to be carefully found, grown, and nurtured. Instead it became readily available at low cost. Suddenly bustling metropolitan cities had fast and cheap supplies of food. This has allowed the human population to skyrocket to more than seven billion people, but the cost to our health is now more glaring than ever.

While it's nice not to have to struggle to attain food, the easy access we enjoy has cheapened our relationship with food. At best, we now look at it purely as a way to eliminate hunger—as if all foods are only meant to get us to the next meal, not to help our body function as it was designed to and to keep us healthy.

This tectonic dietary shift, which took place right in front of our eyes but was far too convenient to cause concern, has warped our intuition about which foods should naturally fill our plates. We are now much too dependent on, and trusting of, what food packages say.

I'm not saying food companies don't care about our health. I'd like to believe that most of them do. But in most areas of our lives, we insist on seeing research, hearing all the sides to each story, and getting second opinions. Yet when it comes to the food we put in our mouths, we often look to the people who *profit* from selling as much of it as possible to us. (To a large extent, their motivation is quantity, not quality.)

Our declining dental health is the perfect red flag of this compromised relationship and blind trust. That's the bad news. The good news is that if we educate ourselves and change our diets, we can regain control over our dental health and, as a result, our overall health.

So what have we forgotten in the past two centuries or so? What *did* our ancestors, who understood food sourcing and preparation in a way that we've forgotten, eat? In order to reset the clock on our health and fulfill our genetic health potential, we must find our way back to this ancient knowledge.

The demons of modern food

It's hard to know exactly what people ate before the agricultural revolution (which is currently thought to have occurred around 10,000 years ago), when we were still hunters and gatherers. But it's estimated that around 72 percent of the foods we eat now are different from the foods people ate back then.[1,2]

These "modern" foods include:

- Sugar
- Grains
- Vegetable oils and refined seed oils
- Processed dairy
- Corn
- Soy

To help you understand why these foods don't contribute to your health, we need to understand how they make their way to our plates in the first place. And why, for the most part, we should avoid them, and eat what people used to eat instead.

SUGAR

Yes, yes, I can hear you saying you know that you shouldn't eat sugar.

Most dentists will tell you that they've been trying to remove sugar from their patients' diets to little or no avail for their entire career. This is a fact around the world: sugar is a difficult subject. Many people who say they don't eat much sugar actually consume far more than they think. And people who admit they eat a lot of sugary foods usually eat an *alarming* amount.

The connection between tooth decay, sugar, and bacteria has been established in scientific literature for a long time, yet the idea of tooth decay does little to dampen our sugar addiction. Nearly everyone knows sugar is bad for them, but they can't stay away from it. Nowadays, it's nearly impossible to go an hour without confronting a sweet snack of some sort. Sugar is one of *the* most consumed products on the planet. We're obsessed with it.

But why is this so? Did we just wake up and all of a sudden find ourselves surrounded by sugar? How did it get to be such an integral part of our lives?

Sweet, addictive, valuable sugar

Thousands of years ago, humans discovered that sugar could be grown as a crop and processed to create a sweet, white powder.[3] Since then, the human psyche has glommed on to sugar with all its might.

Today the world produces more than 170 million metric tons of sugar per year.[4] The average person today has around 20 teaspoons of it every day,[5] but nearly all of my patients eat far more and are unaware of it. Sugar is cheap, tasty, and addictive. Most people can't get enough of it, which is why 74 percent of packaged food contains added sugar.[6] It's also why one of our biggest health challenges is to unwind the viselike grip that sugar has on our lives.

What *is* sugar?

You'll recall that sugars are simple carbohydrates. You'll also remember that in Chapter 5 we talked about how there are fast-metabolizing, harmful strains of bacteria in our bodies that feed off simple sugars or carbs, while the slower-metabolizing bacteria feed off complex carbohydrates, like fiber.

In nature, we simply don't come across simple carbohydrates very often. They're bound up in the fibrous skins of fruit and vegetables. When we eat them with that packaging, we have to break down that fiber, so the sugars are released more slowly and we metabolize them more slowly. But in our modern diet, we come across sugar almost all the time, and it rarely comes with that fiber packaging.

Let's do a (simple) sugar audit of an average day:

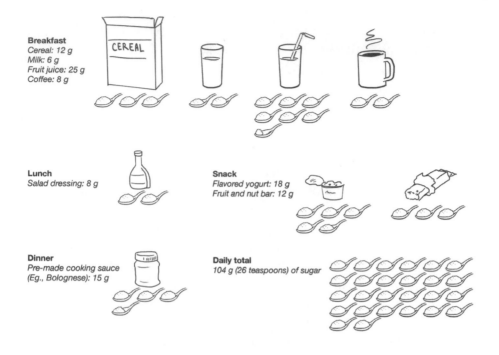

Fig. 20. How sugar sneaks into your daily meals

That's 104 grams (26 teaspoons) of sugar—from foods that would for the most part be considered "healthy." I've found that people *often* consume this much sugar without even beginning to appreciate it.

But if you throw in foods that are *known* to have a lot of sugar, the arithmetic gets even worse:

> *Dessert and sweet snacks:*
>
> Soda 44g
>
> Ice cream 30g
>
> Chocolate bar 26g
>
> Candy 35g

Eat just one of those and your daily sugar intake could be around 130 to 150 grams, or 40 to 45 teaspoons. Eat two of them and you're way over 50 teaspoons.

Think about *that*—a pile of 50 teaspoons of pure sugar. That's how much many of us consume in a single, average day without batting an eyelash.

GRAINS

According to some estimates, humans began eating grains around 23,000 years ago, while others say it could have been as far back as 100,000 years ago.[7]

In any case, most scientists believe that it wasn't until around 10,000 to 14,000 years ago that we began to practice agriculture. That's when grains became a significant part of our diet.

Grains were a logical crop for farmers to focus on. They're edible, highly storable, and can be used to feed livestock. Grains also, of course, are used to make flour, a base for so many of the foods we eat, like bread. Eventually we developed stone mills, which used water or wind to power two large stones to crush the grain. This produced a nutty flour that had all the vitamins, fiber, and other nutrients of the original grain.[8]

At the beginning of the Industrial Revolution in the late 1800s, growing populations created a need for long-lasting flour. So we developed steam mills, which ground grains to a pure white flour, and we removed the fibrous outer bran and germ layers, which could spoil the flour. This made it last longer, but it also robbed the flour of the proteins, fat, vitamins, and other nutrients contained in the original grain. Nevertheless, this processed flour—a starchy carbohydrate with little nutritional benefit beyond raw energy—quickly became a fundamental staple of the modern diet.

Grains and bread today

Today, around 147 million metric tons of wheat is produced every day.[9] And much of it is processed right down into white flour. It's then bleached and treated with chlorine gas as a way to make the gluten proteins mature instantly so the flour is more digestible.

The result is a refined white powder. Remind you of anything? Refined white flour is made up of simple carbs, which the body breaks down into—what else?—sugar.

That's bad news because the vast majority of breads, pastas, and other grain products sold today have a refined white flour base. Even the "whole-grain" varieties available to us are mostly white flour, fortified with B-vitamins, iron, and added fiber. And many other "healthy" packaged foods, like breakfast cereals, white rice, and tortillas, are stuffed with refined white flour. In addition to all the actual sugar we eat, we get a generous second helping from foods we usually don't associate with sugar at all.

Grains are also seeds. In nature, they're meant to be eaten by animals and passed to fresh fertile ground in their feces. They have components that keep them from being broken down in animals' digestive systems. Some of these components, like phytic acids, can cause digestive problems in humans.

Traditional cultures do consume flour, but they generally take great care in growing and nurturing the grain to make sure it retains it nutrients and is digestible. There are three main methods for doing this: soaking, fermenting, and sprouting. Each of them preserves the complex carbs in the grains.

Soaking
Many traditional societies soak their grains before eating them. This neutralizes phytic acid and other substances in the grain that inhibit enzymes that aid digestion. Soaking also adds enzymes that help bring out the grain's nutrients.

Fermenting
In fermentation, bacteria and yeast break down the parts of the grain that are difficult to digest, making it much more edible.

For instance, sourdough bread is created with a "starter" of water and flour and is fermented for several days by adding the yeasts and lactobacilli bacteria that naturally break down the grain.

Sprouting

Sprouting is a traditional way to treat grain that allows it to grow into seedlings, which transforms the indigestible parts of the grain and makes it easier for our bodies to process. Sprouted grains have nutrient profiles closer to those of plants.

Many societies keep their grain seed warm and damp, as it's found in soil. This way, when the seed sprouts, the grain retains more protein, fat, and vitamin B but fewer starchy carbohydrates. With fewer carbs, these grains don't feed as much of the harmful bacteria in our mouth and gut as other grains do. They're also easier to digest.

Are modern grains the cause of gluten intolerance?

Celiac disease is an autoimmune disorder where the body attacks certain cells in the small intestine when it's exposed to gluten—a mix of proteins in wheat, barley, rye, and other grains. Around one million Americans suffer from the disease.[10] The symptoms include digestive problems like diarrhea, bloating, irregular stools, and weight loss, but celiac disease can also cause tooth decay, mouth ulcers, skin allergies, growth problems, irregular periods, and other health issues.

The curious thing is that while human beings have consumed gluten for thousands of years, celiac disease seems to have exploded only in the past 50 years.[11] This puzzles scientists, because there doesn't seem to be a link between gluten tolerance and children who have been exposed—or restricted—from gluten from an early age.[12,13] The disease seems to strike at random.

But when you consider how the majority of grains are now consumed as white flour, it stands to reason that our digestive system has trouble processing gluten when it isn't treated in a way that nurtures its more digestible properties.

Researchers are now learning more about how autoimmunity can be a product of intestinal permeability. When we eat refined flour, our digestive system is flooded with undigested gluten, which triggers an autoimmune reaction that destroys the body's own intestinal cells.

Dr. Alessio Fasano, a gastroenterologist and researcher, has done extensive research on celiac disease that is helping scientists understand how intestinal permeability leads to gluten intolerance. He has found that when people with celiac disease or gluten intolerance eliminate gluten from their diet, which removes the proteins that were passing unchecked through their gut lining, their symptoms subside.[14]

CORN

The United States grows more corn than any other crop. Corn is versatile and cheap, so food manufacturers like to manipulate it and use it as a filler in food. A great many of the packaged products on our supermarket shelves have some form of corn in them—whether it's corn flour, caramel flavor, corn fructose, corn meal, corn oil, corn syrup, dextrin and dextrose, fructose, lactic acid, malt, maltodextrin, mono- and diglycerides, monosodium glutamate, sorbitol, or another variation.

The names of these corn products give them away. They're unnatural—the products of mass-produced, genetically modified crops. They don't contain any of corn's nutritional benefits. And since they're refined and processed down to their simplest elements—much like sugar and flour—our body isn't designed to recognize and digest them.

High-fructose corn syrup

As if plain old sugar didn't cause enough tooth decay on its own, during the 20th century we came up with a new food additive that made sugary products even more lethal. It seems like you can find it in every mass-produced food that's at all sweet. It's called high-fructose corn syrup, and it's like sugar on steroids.

Isolated from cornstarch, high-fructose corn syrup is industrially processed so that some of its glucose becomes fructose, which is much sweeter than normal sugar. High-fructose corn syrup lets food companies sweeten their foods more cost-effectively.

But what's good for food manufacturers is bad for our mouths and bodies. Eating a diet high in fructose adds a metabolic wild card to our system that begins with tooth decay and ends with organs that are drowning in sugar. High blood sugar can interfere with teeth and bone formation,[15] and high-fructose corn syrup causes higher blood sugar swings than normal sugar does. And while all of our cells can metabolize glucose for energy, we can metabolize fructose only in our liver, where it causes inflammation. It also leads to weight gain and other health issues.[16]

In nature, fructose is at its highest availability from fruits in fall as they ripen and drop to the ground. Our bodies are designed to eat them right then, so they can store the excess sugar as fat and insulation around our organs during the cold winter. Our bodies aren't meant to consume an excess of fructose all yearround.

PROCESSED VEGETABLE OILS

While many people are familiar with the dangers of sugar and processed grains, processed or refined vegetable oils also carry important health risks.

To a large degree, these processed vegetable oils have replaced the natural fats in our diet. Food companies and consumers love refined, polyunsaturated oils—like corn, canola, and sunflower oil—because they are cheap to manufacture and are easy to store and transport.

The problem is that the polyunsaturated fats in these oils are artificially extracted through a high heat chemical process called hydrogenation. The exposure to high temperatures makes them *highly* reactive. They can become very unstable in our bodies, causing inflammation. Cooking polyunsaturated oils on high heat can also turn them into partially hydrogenated fats, also known as trans fats. Trans fats, which tend to show up in snack foods and fast food, can further harm our cells and blood and increase the risk of heart attack.[17]

The rise of refined oils

How did processed, or refined, oils become so popular? For the most part, it all began with margarine.

Margarine

In 1831, Emperor Napoleon III of France wanted a butter alternative suitable to feed the armed forces and the lower classes. Chemist Hippolyte Mège-Mouriès answered the call. He developed a way to hydrogenate vegetable oil, which turned it into a solid compound that could potentially replace butter. Margarine was born.[18]

Margarine didn't have quite the same taste or color as butter. Initially it was met with resistance. But during the Great Depression and World War II, the world's butter supply was greatly restricted and margarine became more widely accepted. Processed, hydrogenated fats were already relatively cheap and easy to produce. Now they were popular. A trend was born: margarine showed that we could replace natural fats with fats made in a chemistry lab.

Cottonseed Oil (Crisco)

In 1911, Procter & Gamble started selling hydrogenated cottonseed oil as a cooking fat under the name Crisco, as in "crystallized cottonseed oil."[19]

Today's Crisco no longer contains cottonseed oil. But since it's so inexpensive, restaurants still use cottonseed oil for frying, and it's found in countless packaged foods—everything from nut spreads to cereals to health bars.

Canola Oil

In the late 1970s, Canadian plant breeders figured out how to genetically modify a variety of rapeseed (a relative of mustard) to produce a new monounsaturated oil. They hoped it could be a healthy alternative to polyunsaturated oils. "Rapeseed oil" wasn't exactly the most marketable name, so the industry christened it "canola oil," short for "Canadian oil." At the time, rapeseed was grown mainly in Canada.[20]

Canola oil now sits in the pantry or kitchen of millions of homes around the world. The research on it is mixed, and there aren't many long-term studies on it. Animal studies, however, have shown an association between rapeseed oil and fibrotic lesions of the heart.[21] Considering how little we really know about it and the track record of other refined seed oils, I recommend that my patients stay away from canola oil entirely.

Soybean oil

Soybean oil, like other refined vegetable oils, is unhealthy. The same goes for soy milk and other soy products. Soy products are generally treated with a high-heat extraction process to remove the oils from the beans. Then they're highly modified with chemical processes before they become the products you see on supermarket shelves. All of this changes their compounds, making them less recognizable to our bodies.

When you see the word *soy* on a package, it's tempting to think automatically that it's healthy. But the chemical processes it's likely been through make it just as refined as the other food products we've been talking about. Of course, not all soy products are harmful. Soy has been used as an ingredient in food by traditional cultures for a very long time. For instance, many Asian cultures ferment it to turn it into bean curd and used in foods such as traditional tofu or tempeh. Unlike processing it or adding a lot of heat to it, fermenting soybeans is an excellent way to preserve its nutritional properties.

DAIRY

Since humans began to domesticate animals, societies around the world have consumed dairy products from the milk of cows, sheep, goats, camels, and other animals.

Lactose is a type of sugar found in milk. It's made up of two simple carbohydrates, glucose and galactose. Because of this different chemical make-up from other sugars, your digestive system needs a special enzyme called lactase to digest it.

Young children almost universally produce lactase and can digest the lactose in their mother's milk. But some people don't have lactase persistence, or the ability to produce lactase in adulthood. Approximately 65 percent of the human population has a reduced ability to consume lactose after the age of about seven or eight.[22]

Human beings also became the only species who consume other animals' milk. It all began 11,000 years ago, as farming blossomed in the Middle East. Around that time, cattle herders learned how to ferment milk to make cheese or yogurt, which had lactose levels the human body could process.[23]

Thousands of years later, around 7,500 B.C., one of the most recent and profound examples of epigenetics occurred. As humans moved into the Northern European climate, the lack of sun increased the need to consume dairy products containing vitamin D. Gradual epigenetic changes led to a genetic mutation that spread through Europe and gave adults the ability to produce the lactase enzyme. This let them drink milk throughout their lives.

The culture around dairy

For thousands of years, people drank milk mainly from local cows that were milked by hand. But industrialization changed all that. Local farms couldn't supply enough milk to feed cities, so milk and dairy became an industry itself.[24]

By 1914, Louis Pasteur's method of heating a liquid and then cooling it to kill any pathogens in it—otherwise known as pasteurization—had become standard practice among American dairy producers. This expanded milk's shelf life and it could be shipped long distances. People could now get milk basically whenever they wanted it.[25]

But this convenience came at a hidden cost.

Pasteurization and homogenized dairy

Cow's milk contains special fatty acid droplets that are designed to deliver crucial vitamins and minerals to calves. Meanwhile, cow's udders are filled with bacteria, specifically lactobacillus. So when milk comes out of the udder, it contains a healthy package of fatty acids, vitamins, minerals, and bacteria. The digestive tract—whether it's in a cow or a person—depends on these bacteria to properly digest the milk and make use of its nutrients.[26]

But pasteurization kills a large number of these bacteria, and it also bakes the casein proteins that make up around 80 percent of the protein in milk.[27] This baking warps the structure of the caseins, making them harder for us to digest.

Milk that comes out of a cow is uneven in color and consistency because the cream in it tends to rise to the top. Natural milk wouldn't look so good on supermarket shelves for that reason, so dairy companies homogenize it.

Homogenization is a process in which milk is squeezed through tiny metal shafts at high heat to "flatten" its fat particles and make its color and consistency uniform. The problem is that the process squeezes the fatty acids, which are the tails of the fat molecules. Fats behave the way they do because of the shape and size of their tail. When you change the tail of a fatty acid, you change its behavior as a molecule, which makes it harder for our body to process it.

If you think back to Chapter 5, you'll recall the incredibly important role that bacteria play in our digestion, gut lining, and immune system. Now, when you think about how much we've changed the environments of cows and the makeup of their milk, and how much we've manipulated our own microbiome, our modern problems with dairy explain themselves.

HOW MODERN FARMING CHANGES THE MEAT THAT YOU EAT

Grass-fed versus grain-fed cattle

Today we eat more meat than ever, but we've severely compromised the quality of that meat.

We used to eat animals that grew up in their natural habitat and lived on natural foods like grass. Then, during World War II, farmers produced more grain than the American population could consume, and they started feeding the surplus grain to their cattle. They soon discovered that feeding cattle a diet based on grain fattened them up for slaughter more quickly. Seventy-five years ago, it took a cow four or five years to grow big enough for slaughter. Today, by feeding them grains like corn and giving them protein supplements, anti-bloating medications, and growth hormone, cattle can be slaughtered at just 14 to 16 months of age.[28]

To make matters worse, corn-fed cattle are susceptible to many illnesses, so dairy producers continually give them antibiotics, which lead them to develop antibiotic-resistant bacteria, which increasingly render modern medicine ineffective.[29]

Vitamins and minerals in beef

If you're a steak lover, you're probably familiar with the term "marbled meat." Today we even grade meat based on its level of marbling. But what many people don't appreciate is that the "marble" in meat is really fat that's dispersed within the muscle.

While the marbling in grain-fed beef is white, the fat in grass-fed beef is usually a yellow-gray color. The yellow is from the carotenoids (vitamin A precursors) the animal absorbs by eating grass. The fat in grain-fed beef is generally lower in fat-soluble vitamins A and E. It also contains fewer minerals, like zinc, iron, and phosphorus.[30] And its omega fatty acids are skewed; it has fewer omega-3 fats and more omega-6 fats, which increase inflammation in the body.[31]

ANCESTRAL EATING—GOING BACK TO THE BASICS

Weston Price highlighted the robust dental and bodily health of the traditional or native societies he studied, which he attributed to their traditional diets. Some might call this *ancestral eating.*

The Dental Diet is about contextualizing the food that sits on our plate today so we can make choices that bring our diet closer to those traditional—and healthier—ideals.

People sometimes think ancestral eating is all about eating the foods that cavemen ate. Today it's very difficult to compare our diet to Paleolithic times. Many of the foods that ancient humans ate back then simply aren't available today or have evolved to become significantly different (for example, the fruit that hunter-gatherers ate was much more fibrous than the fruit we eat today).[32] And besides, until the Industrial Revolution, none of these changes led to any serious degeneration in our health. Not only is it impossible to go back to that caveman/ancestral model of eating, it's also unnecessary.

Today, you don't need to eat a strictly traditional, or native, or ancestral diet, but you need to understand the principles behind the foods our ancient forebears did eat, because their nutritional patterns were developed and honed before the Industrial Revolution brought us the processed, problematic foods I've described above. These diets aren't based on mass production, long shelf life, or any of the other commercial priorities our modern foods are developed around. Instead, they're based on food as it's naturally found in the environment, and on our own health.

Whole foods versus refined foods

Traditional societies needed to make sure that every resource in their food supply was exploited, because supplies weren't unlimited like they are today. Fittingly, our bodies are designed to pull nutrients from all the different parts of plants and animals, not just select parts of them. The more of the plant we eat, and the more of the animal we eat, the more nutrients we get.

Think about how animals live in the wild. When they come across an edible plant or a smaller/weaker animal, wild animals usually eat the entire organism. At the very least, they consume more of it than we'd think to eat.

Traditional diets have long been centered on providing these nutrients in their natural form. These include natural, unprocessed full fats from animals and whole plants. Traditional societies around the world have used every part of the living creature in order to provide their bodies with these nutrients for tens of thousands of years.

Here are some examples of full-fat foods that traditional diets valued for many thousands of years.

- Ghee
- Raw butter and raw cream from grass-fed cows
- Tallow and suet from grass-finished cows, bison, elk, and other ruminant animals
- Lard from pasture-raised pigs
- Fat from pasture-raised ducks, geese, and chickens
- Whole fish and seafood, and fats including cod-liver oil
- Unrefined coconut oil, palm kernel oil, and unrefined, cold-pressed, extra-virgin olive oil.

Both traditional cultures and wild animals alike have focused on eating the organs of an animal, such as the liver. As we talked about earlier, the organs are the richest sources of those all-important fat-soluble vitamins A, D, and K2, which allow us to build and maintain strong bones.

Traditional diets nearly unanimously include cuts of meats that are good sources of fat-soluble vitamins. These include organ meats, also known as offal meats, like liver, stomachs, intestines, hearts, and brains.

To name a few examples, the Chinese eat dim sum dishes featuring wobbly cubes of coagulated duck blood and cow tripe laced with shredded ginger. Italians eat organ meat called *pajata*, the milk-containing intestines of an unweaned calf. And Pakistanis eat *kat-a-kat*, which is a hash of kidney, heart, brain, liver, and testicles of goats or sheep.

THE IMPORTANCE OF FOOD PREPARATION

We should note that eating for a healthy mouth and body is not only a matter of picking the right foods. If you want to get the right amount of fat-soluble vitamins and other key nutrients into your diet, the way your food is prepared is just as crucial.

Fermented foods

In fermentation, bacteria convert sugars to alcohol, acids, or carbon dioxide—compounds that are more stable and last longer. Fermentation happens all the time in nature, thanks to organisms like yeast and bacteria. But of course humans have for a long time known how to use it to their advantage as well.

Fermentation is a great way of preserving foods that, for one reason or another, aren't available year-round, like fresh vegetables. So fermented foods played prominent roles in traditional diets.

Europeans have long eaten fermented dairy, cabbage (sauerkraut), grape leaves, herbs, and root vegetables. Indians consume lassi as a predinner yogurt drink. In Bulgaria, people stay healthy by consuming raw fermented milk and kefir. Chinese workers ate acid-fermented vegetables while building the Great Wall. Centuries ago, the Koreans developed kimchi by acid-fermenting cabbage and other vegetables. Today, across various Asian countries, people eat all kinds of pickled vegetables. And African cultures still routinely use lactic acid fermentation as a way of preserving crops like corn.[33]

Some fermented foods still have a prominent place in our modern diet, though many of us don't realize that. Cheese and yogurt are made from fermented milk. Wine is fermented grapes. Pickles are fermented cucumbers.

Fermented foods tend to be great for our health because the fermentation process produces valuable nutrients, including vitamins like thiamine, nicotinic acid, biotin, riboflavin, and the very valuable K2 vitamin. Grains are much more digestible and nutritious after they've been fermented.

But our modern, processed foods have generally been robbed

147

of the nutrients we need to keep our mouths and bodies balanced and healthy.

Broths

Broths or soup stocks cooked with animal bones have been a staple of human diets around the world for thousands of years.

The beauty of a broth is that it's full of minerals and nutrients and is an excellent source of gelatin (made from denatured collagen), which helps build bones, cartilage, and skin. Broths are a fundamental part of any diet designed around the health of our mouth, digestive system, joints, and skeletal system.

Broths used to be a much bigger part of people's diets, whether they consumed them in soups, stews, gravies, or other hot, liquid-based dishes. But they've faded from our diet in favor of mass-produced, nutrient-deficient alternatives like canned soups and frozen meals.

BE A FOOD DETECTIVE

Sugar is still the primary culprit in tooth decay. But we have to understand that our modern diet is filled with unnatural foods that can damage our mouths and bodies in other ways. I hope this chapter has given you a lens for looking at food that will help you distinguish natural food from harmful simulations of it.

Once you get in the habit of looking at food through this new lens, it will be hard to justify eating something that you know your body won't recognize. Your natural instincts will take you back to foods that you *are* meant to eat. Your diet will begin to align with the foods your ancestors ate. And your mouth and your body will thank you for it.

CHAPTER 8

FROM LOW-FAT TO CHOLESTEROL

How We're Recommending Sickness

It's hard to picture this now, but it wasn't so long ago that doctors were endorsing certain brands of cigarettes. As late as 1949, Camel ran magazine ads that pictured a man in a white coat and the words "More doctors smoke Camels than any other cigarette."

Even then, the medical community—if not the public at large—knew that cigarettes weren't necessarily *healthy*. But the fact that doctors used to put their names behind certain brands shows you how much medical knowledge can evolve in the span of a single lifetime. What you were taught as a child might be proven false by the time you're an adult.

One of the hardest challenges I have as a dentist is to reverse people's ingrained beliefs about what's healthy. It all starts off okay. When I say, "You need to change your diet to protect your mouth's health," they usually nod in agreement. If I tell them their children have to eat differently to protect their mouths, they understand.

But it all comes to a grinding halt when I explain that a healthy diet includes eating foods with more fat than they're used to. Their expression immediately changes, as if to say, "Won't that make me *gain weight* and *put me at risk of a heart attack?*" Fat is universally known as a menace to your arteries. It's a challenge to convince people that fat can help keep you healthy, and even help keep you thin.

Like any of the compounds that come in the foods we eat, fats serve a definite purpose in our bodies. Among other things, they make up the membranes of our cells that keep them flexible and strong. Yet everyone reading this book is probably familiar with the idea that the less fat you eat, the healthier you'll be— and that in order to lose weight the "right" way, you have to eat low-fat foods. It's an idea that's overwhelmingly advanced by doctors, dieticians, and the media.

You can tell how widely accepted this is just by taking a look at the shelves in your local supermarket. Low-fat foods tend to enjoy prominent placement, and their packaging almost always highlights that they're low-fat. Marketers would never hide that characteristic.

Yet, paradoxically, even though we're more aware than ever of the supposed benefits of low-fat dieting, the problems that it had aimed to stop are far worse than when they were first recommended. In 2014, the World Health Organization estimated that 1.9 billion adults worldwide were overweight. Of these, more than 600 million were obese.[1]

There have been countless studies on this, books written about it, and more than enough finger-pointing to go around. But very few have looked at how obesity and weight problems can be linked back to our mouth. Tooth decay, obesity, heart disease, and other chronic illnesses are all driven by the same basic nutritional factors, so it stands to reason that eating to take care of the teeth and mouth automatically helps protect against those other diseases.

THE BIRTH OF "LOW FAT"

In the 1940s, a physiologist named Ancel Keys tried to find out why middle-aged American men were suffering from a relatively high rate of heart attacks.

Keys did a long-term study on business executives from Minnesota aged 45 to 55. He tracked their blood pressure, cholesterol, diet, and other lifestyle factors. These men ate a lot of meat and dairy foods that were high in saturated fat, which led Keys to develop his famous lipid–heart hypothesis.[2] It stated that eating foods high in saturated fats raised the level of harmful cholesterol in the blood and increased the risk of heart disease and stroke.

To further test his theory, Keys carried out his Seven Countries Study, in which he looked at the rates of heart disease and the diets of middle-aged men in seven countries around the world. The study seemed to confirm his earlier conclusions, but there's strong evidence that he cherry-picked the data to validate his ideas.[3]

In time, the low-fat ideal became fully baked into the Western world's dietary consciousness—and, really, *conscience*—which has led to sweeping changes in the way we eat and think about food and nutrition.

We aim to eat as few calories as we can, rather than to consume as many *nutrients* as we can. We shun foods that are high in fat, even when they're high in many other things our bodies need. We confuse *looking* like we're in shape on the outside with actually *being* in shape on the inside.

MISCONCEPTIONS ABOUT SATURATED FAT, CHOLESTEROL, AND HEART DISEASE

In 1977 the U.S. Senate Select Committee on Nutrition and Human Needs endorsed the lipid–heart hypothesis. In 1980 the U.S. government published the first version of its *Dietary Guidelines for Americans*, in which it told us to eat more fruits, vegetables, grains, and poultry, and to substitute whole-fat animal and dairy products for their leaner versions.[4]

What's often missed, however, is that the original report and those that have come since have also been criticized by scientists who say that more research is needed to come to such definitive conclusions.[5]

Since then, the low-fat movement has shaped our zeitgeist of "healthy eating." Nearly all patients I speak to feel about fat the same way they feel about bacteria—that it's uniformly bad. So before I explain why fat is actually good for us, I'd like to wipe the slate clean of your preconceptions. Let's go over some of the more popular, and powerful, myths about fat and why they're inaccurate.

1. **Low-fat diets protect against heart disease, obesity, and diabetes:** *Unproven*

    Sixty years have passed since the low-fat movement began, so we now have a lot of data that let us measure its effect on society's overall health.

    Between 1980 and 2000, deaths linked to heart disease did decrease.[6] But this may have been due to improvements in surgery and medicine more than anything else. Today heart disease is still the leading cause of death for both men and women. Obesity rates are increasing—44 percent of the U.S. population could be obese by 2030.[7] And even more compellingly, type 2 diabetes has appeared almost out of nowhere since the 1970s.[8]

2. **Saturated fats cause heart disease:** *False*

    The first and most significant assumption of the low-fat movement is the lipid–heart hypothesis, which posits that saturated fat leads to heart disease. In 2010, a large study showed that there actually is no link between heart disease and saturated fat.[9]

    In fact, a more recent 2014 study showed that a saturated fat found in dairy, called margaric acid, "significantly reduced" the risk of heart disease, while two kinds of saturated fat found in palm oil and animal products had only a "weak link" to heart disease.[10] It also illuminated how existing data indicate that so-called heart-healthy polyunsaturated fats, like sunflower oil, have no positive effect on the risk of heart disease—more evidence of how little we've understood about how fat interacts with our bodies.

3. **High blood cholesterol leads to heart disease:** *False*

For years, health experts have recommended that we avoid foods high in cholesterol because they increase the risk of heart disease. Increased levels of low-density lipoprotein cholesterol (LDL cholesterol, also known as "bad" cholesterol) were believed to lead to an increased risk of heart attack.

But more recent studies published by the *American Heart Journal* show that most people hospitalized for a heart attack *don't* have cholesterol levels that would medically indicate that they were at a high risk for a heart attack.[11] Theses studies imply that our long-held assumptions about blood cholesterol and heart disease, "validated" by the low-fat movement, were never based in reality.

4. **Saturated fats raise bad cholesterol:** *False*

The lipid–heart hypothesis also assumes that dietary saturated fats raise LDL, the "bad" blood cholesterol. But research has now clearly shown that eating dietary saturated fats not only does *not* shift the proportion of LDL cholesterols in the blood, but actually helps LDL particles gain density and become "good" cholesterol (high-density lipoprotein cholesterol, or HDL).[12,13]

5. **Dietary cholesterol raises blood cholesterol:** *False*

Dietary cholesterol—the cholesterol contained in the food we eat—was long thought to raise the level of the cholesterol in our blood, which can be the bad kind or the good kind. But studies have found that while people respond differently to dietary cholesterol, consuming it in and of itself doesn't change levels of blood cholesterol.[14] In other words, contrary to what we previously assumed, cholesterol from food doesn't directly translate to higher HDL or LDL readings in the blood.

HOW THE LOW-FAT MOVEMENT STOLE OUR HEARTS

The power of hindsight is one thing. But you may be wondering why, if all of these assumptions about the benefits of a low-fat diet are wrong, did we accept them in the first place?

In truth, the lipid–heart hypothesis was always just that: a hypothesis. The scientific evidence that supposedly proved it correct was always considered controversial. But it still became enshrined in federal public health policy and was promoted by health care practitioners and the media. How did that happen? We were swept up in a perfect storm fueled by our growing desire for an answer to heart disease and a societal preference for taut, slim "bikini bodies."

By the mid-eighties, there was an overwhelming consensus that the low-fat diet was appropriate not only for high-risk patients, but also as a preventive measure against heart disease for everyone else except babies.[15]

(Let's stop to think about that for a second. The idea that babies need a diet *different* from that of adults is absurd. The reality is that babies and adults need the same things, just in different amounts.)

In the 1980s, food producers realized that the low-fat movement was an opportunity for new profits and revenue streams. The industry began replacing natural foods with processed alternatives that were largely stripped of saturated fats. But this led to another problem: taking the fat out made most of these foods taste less appealing. So to put flavor back in, the industry packed them with sugar and refined polyunsaturated oils. In the 1990s, this became known as the "Snackwell's phenomenon,"[16] named after the Nabisco line of snacks that were low-fat but packed with carbohydrates and calories.

THE TRUTH ABOUT THE MEDITERRANEAN DIET

Today one of the most universally accepted "models" of a healthy diet is the Mediterranean diet. The notion itself came from Ancel Keys. The Mediterranean diet, as Keys interpreted it, was low in saturated fats and based on whole fish, seafood, olive oil, lots of vegetables, and well-treated whole grains. (Italians are meticulous with their pasta and dough practices.) For the most part, a diet consisting of these foods is healthy. But Keys's interpretation of the Mediterranean diet left out some key food groups and was not a *completely* authentic representation.

When you take a look at what people in Italy actually eat, it might clear up why the "true" Mediterranean diet should *not* be looked at as a low-fat diet. In fact, foods rich in fat-soluble vitamins, including saturated fat, are at the center of the real Mediterranean diet.

Italy is a large country covering vastly different geographical regions, with many different subcultures. Because of this wide geographical spread, there's really no single form of "Italian cuisine." Nevertheless, it's fair to make some generalizations about traditional Italian cooking. Some of the most famous dishes in Italian cooking are based on foods rich in saturated fat, including butter, cheese (from both goats and cows), fatty cuts of meat, organ meats, and seafood high in saturated fat.[17] Let's take a quick look at these dishes and see if they fit the ideal of the Mediterranean diet that we're conditioned to picture in our minds.

Cured meats

Italian cuisine is famous for its cured meats, called *salumi*. There's *capicola*, which is made from the neck or shoulder of a pig, and *soppressata*, made from pressed pork belly, tongue, stomach, and other parts of the pig. There's also *pancetta,* a salt-cured and spiced meat made from the belly of the pig, and *lardo*, which is made from the back fat of a pig and is usually cured with rosemary. And there are plenty of other examples of salumi. But none of them are low-fat.

Organs and fatty cuts of meat

Italian cooking also contains a variety of dishes that use offal and organ meats, including chicken liver pâté and calf's liver with onions. In *cucina povera,* Italian peasant cooking, dishes based on organ meats, like sautéed lamb offal, are quite popular.

One of the most common street foods in central Italy is *porchetta,* a whole roasted pig, which is often carved up from snout to toe for sandwiches or for people to take home. And there's mackerel, a fish eaten in many Italian regions that has a relatively high amount of saturated fat.

Eggs

For a long time, we thought egg yolks were unhealthy because they're high in cholesterol. But they're also a staple of Italian cooking, the most notable egg dish being the *frittata*, a sort of omelet made from 8 to 10 eggs and filled with various vegetables, cheeses, and meats. (As discussed above, we now know that eating foods that contain high amounts of cholesterol in fact does *not* raise blood cholesterol. Frittata fans rejoice.)

Full-fat milk and cheeses

The three most important cheeses in Italian cooking are each high in saturated fat. You'll almost certainly recognize their names.

Parmigiano-Reggiano is made from raw cow's milk; the hard, nutty cheese is aged for two to three years. *Mozzarella* is made from Italian buffalo milk. *Ricotta* is made from whey from cow, sheep, goat, or buffalo milk. In *The Blue Zones*, Dan Buettner, a National Geographic Fellow and author, notes that some of the longest-living Italians are found in Sardinia, where they drink raw goat's milk high in fat and fat-soluble vitamins.

In the West, we've largely learned the wrong lessons from the Mediterranean diet. The irony is that the real Mediterranean diet closely resembles the diets of the traditional societies that Weston Price described—diets based on whole foods that were full-fat and rich in fat-soluble vitamins. The low-fat, processed-food diet that we've long held up as ideal is the *antithesis* of these traditional eating models.

WHY DO WE NEED FATS? WHAT DO THEY DO?

Saturated and unsaturated fats

The foods we eat have mixes of saturated and unsaturated fatty acids in them. These two types of fat complement each other in nature, and since we're part of nature ourselves, they are complementary in our bodies as well. There is no one-size-fits-all answer for how much of each fat we should eat. The bottom line is that, like the other nutrients we've talked about in this book and like most things in life, we need a balance of saturated and unsaturated fats to be at peak health.

They're particularly important to our cell membranes. Our cells are surrounded by thousands, if not millions, of foreign molecules at any given time. So they need a protective skin that is permeable enough to let friendly compounds in but impermeable enough to keep unwanted compounds out. The cell membrane is that protective skin.

Saturated fats are not very reactive; in fact, they're actually some of the most stable compounds we take in. And they help give the cell membranes a sort of stability or structural integrity—they help keep them rigid. Unsaturated fats, on the other hand, help keep the membrane more fluid and flexible, which is necessary for the cell to travel and to exchange the compounds it needs to take in or expel.

For these same reasons, saturated and unsaturated fats are also vital to immune cells and the many signaling hormones that control them. Suffice it to say that fats are important to our health in countless ways.

The different types of fats, and what they do in the body

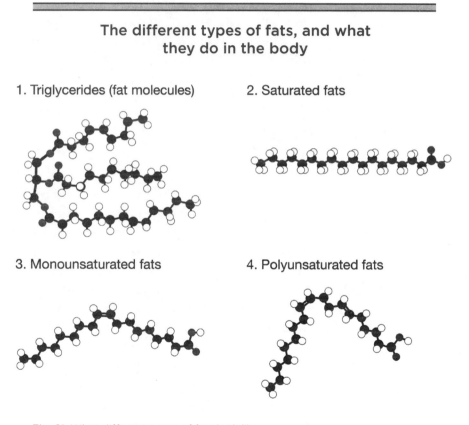

1. Triglycerides (fat molecules)

2. Saturated fats

3. Monounsaturated fats

4. Polyunsaturated fats

Fig. 21. What different types of fats look like

I'd like to talk to you about what fat actually does in our bodies. But to understand that, we first need to understand the structure of fats themselves:

Lipid is a general term for fats and oils. If a lipid is solid at room temperature, it's called fat. If it's liquid at room temperature, it's oil. The ability of fats to be both a liquid and a solid make them very handy assets for the bodies' cells.

Fat molecules (also called triglycerides) consist of three fatty acid chains, comprised of strings of carbon atoms that are each bonded with hydrogen atoms and attached to a monoglyceride—a simple compound of hydrogen and oxygen atoms.

In nature, all fats are either saturated or unsaturated. It all depends on the carbon atoms that make up the fatty acid chains.

In **saturated fats**, the carbon and hydrogen molecules in the fatty acid chains are all joined by single bonds. No other molecules can join the chain because all the bonds are "in use." They're maxed out, or "saturated."

Since they're maxed out, less reactive, and more stable, saturated fats tend to be solids at body temperatures and have higher melting points. They're mainly found in animal products, like beef, poultry, and dairy products, including hard cheeses (such as cheddar), whole milk, cream, butter, lard, tallow, ghee, suet, palm oil, and coconut oil.

In **unsaturated fats**, the carbon molecules in the fatty acid chains have at least one double bond. When two molecules are attached by a double bond, another molecule *can* potentially link up with them. They're not maxed out; they're "unsaturated."

Due to their double bond, unsaturated fats are more reactive and fluid and have lower melting points. They're usually liquids at room temperature.

Unsaturated fats come in two forms: monounsaturated and polyunsaturated.

Monounsaturated fats have fatty acid chains that contain one double bond. Olive oil, peanut oils, and avocados are sources of monounsaturated fat.

Polyunsaturated fats have fatty acid chains that contain multiple double bonds. Their higher number of double bonds makes them more reactive than monounsaturated fats. Common sources of polyunsaturated fat are fatty fish, safflower, sesame and sunflower seeds, corn, soybeans, and many nuts and seeds and their oils.

It's misleading to look at fats in isolation because nature intended to them to fit *together*, like pieces in a puzzle.

Our cell membranes, for instance, need a mix of saturated, monounsaturated, and polyunsaturated fatty acids to be stable, flexible, and healthy overall. This is why we must eat fats in their natural state—so that we get all the pieces to the puzzle.

"Good" and "bad" fats

Right now you might be thinking: *Wait a second, I know all fats aren't bad. There are some bad fats, but there are also those good fats we hear so much about.* The concept of "good fats" and "bad fats" evolved out of the lipid–heart hypothesis. Unfortunately, it's caused more confusion than clarity.

For the most part, the idea came from a study carried out in the 1970s by Danish scientists who investigated the Inuit people of Greenland. They noted the low incidence of heart disease among these native people, who ate large amounts of whale blubber, seal oil, and fish.[18] The scientists concluded that the Inuits' native diet was good for heart health. Blubber and seal oil are rich in omega-3 fats, and the researchers believed that omega-3s were the Inuits' secret weapon against heart disease.

While whale blubber and seal oil are rich in omega-3s, they also contain relatively high amounts of saturated fats. Thanks to Ancel Keys, the scientific community already believed saturated fats were uniformly bad for heart health. In 2002 it was announced by heart foundations that polyunsaturated fats like omega-3s had to be uniformly good for heart health.[19] That's how polyunsaturated fats (mistakenly) got their "good fat" moniker.

The reality is that in nature, fats don't exist in isolation. On the chemical level, fats like to band together with other types of fats, which means that saturated, monounsaturated, and polyunsaturated fats tend to all come in a package. Omega-3 supplements have not been confirmed to have either positive or negative effect on heart disease.[20] Singling out *one* type of fat as healthy or "good" ignores this. Fats are healthy only when they come in that complete, balanced package, which includes fat-soluble vitamins nicely bundled with natural fats.

Omega-3 and omega-6 fatty acids

There are two kinds of polyunsaturated fats that we come across more than any others: omega-3s and omega-6s. They're also known as "essential fatty acids" because we get them only from food we eat; our bodies can't manufacture them.

Like other fats, omega-3 and omega-6 fatty acids help with cell membrane, brain, and hormone function. But they're particularly crucial for regulating inflammation in the body.

Omega-3s are anti-inflammatory agents. They are found in plants like flax, hemp, and chia; in fish and fish oils; and in some egg and dairy products.

Omega-6 fatty acids enable inflammation. They're found in nuts and seeds, including sesame seeds, pumpkin seeds, walnuts, pine nuts, Brazil nuts, pecans, peanuts, and almonds. They're also found in refined oils like sunflower, corn, and cottonseed oils.

In nature, omega-3s and omega-6s naturally exist in a 1:1 ratio. But today we consume much more of the inflammation-enabling omega-6s than we do of the anti-inflammatory omega-3s. By some estimates, this ratio is a perilous 16:1.[21]

Lipoproteins and "good" and "bad" cholesterol

We've already discussed "good" and "bad" cholesterol. Those labels refer to LDL and HDL lipoproteins, which together constitute our blood cholesterol. What are lipoproteins? Think of them as very tiny, very clever packages that let our body transport fats.

Your body is more than 60 percent water, which is a great medium for delivering things. But because our system is water based, fats and fat-soluble substances like some vitamins and cholesterol don't travel well inside us on their own. (It's literally mixing oil and water.) To get the fats and fat-soluble compounds to your teeth and the other structures that need them, they need a sort of coating or packaging that is *water*-soluble. That's where the lipoproteins come in.

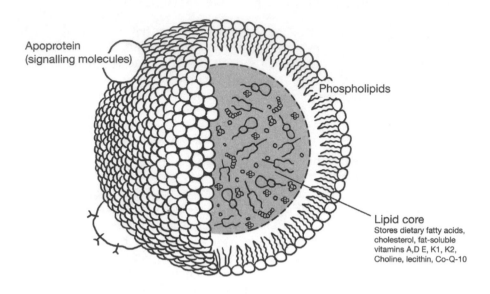

Apoprotein
(signalling molecules)

Phospholipids

Lipid core
Stores dietary fatty acids,
cholesterol, fat-soluble
vitamins A,D E, K1, K2,
Choline, lecithin, Co-Q-10

Fig. 22. Lipoproteins: the carriers of fat-soluble substances through the body

Lipoproteins are packages of fats, cholesterol, and fat-soluble nutrients, all put together in one handy particle that travels easily in our blood. Much like the outside of a UPS package, the protein coating of a lipoprotein essentially contains an "address." The lipoprotein travels through the blood until it gets to a cell that matches with that address. The cell takes in the lipoprotein and begins to use the nutrients inside.

The body also uses lipoproteins to transport fatty substances from cells to the liver and from the liver back to cells. To do this, the body uses cycles of higher-density (HDL) and lower-density (LDL) lipoproteins. HDLs are *generally* produced and released from the liver. The body uses HDLs and LDLs in different ways—and needs both.

Doctors know that certain LDL particles can stick to the walls of our arteries and form dangerous plaques. That's why LDL is considered to be the bad cholesterol. And since HDLs don't get caught in arteries and can help break up clusters of LDL particles, flush them from the arteries, and bring them to the liver, HDL is known as the good cholesterol. But this distinction is misleading. Our body needs both HDLs and LDLs to work together to form our fat-packaging system.

Cholesterol in our bodies versus cholesterol in our food

The National Institutes of Health define cholesterol as "a waxy, fat-like substance that's found in all cells of the body." The NIH goes on to say that "your body needs cholesterol to make hormones, vitamin D, and substances that help you digest foods."[22] Lipoproteins are made up of cholesterol and the other types of fats. Seventy-five percent of the cholesterol in our bodies is produced by the liver; the other twenty-five percent comes from the foods we eat.[23]

When we talk about a person's blood cholesterol levels, or HDL and LDL levels, we're referring to their blood (or serum) cholesterol—the amount *in* their bloodstream.[24] We're not talking about the amount of cholesterol in the food they *eat*. That's an important distinction, because we used to think—and feel quite certain, really—that the cholesterol in the food we ate raised the level of the cholesterol in our blood. That's why we all thought we shouldn't eat too many eggs, for instance. But our bodies actually need dietary cholesterol to digest fats and carry all of the fat-soluble substances in lipoproteins.

◆ ◆ ◆

HOW UNNATURAL FOODS STARVE YOUR TEETH OF KEY NUTRIENTS

We have now discussed how important the fat-soluble vitamins are for the health of our teeth, bones, and organs and how they travel through our body with the help of lipoproteins. When our lipoprotein delivery system is off-balance, our teeth, bones, and tissues can't get all the fat-soluble vitamins they need. That's why a diet low in saturated fats and cholesterol stands a good chance of clogging our arteries and putting us at risk of heart disease just the same.

Processed oils deprive us of fat-soluble vitamins as well, in more ways than one. First, refined, polyunsaturated oils don't contain *any* fat-soluble vitamins. Even worse, the fats in them are highly unstable and are likely to damage lipoproteins that are designed to carry them. So when we consume them, we're not only starving our fat-soluble vitamin delivery system of the very materials it's supposed to deliver. We're also damaging the postal system itself.

Unfortunately, most of the fats in our diet now come from refined vegetable and other cooking oils mainly composed of polyunsaturated fats. And a lot of our junk food still contains partially hydrogenated fats, or trans fats, which can distort our cell membranes; create chaos in our blood, tissues, and organs; and lead to inflammation and heart disease.[25]

At the same time, we've increasingly been turning away from saturated fats, which are contained in more natural foods, like butter. So we're basically moving away from the natural balance of saturated and unsaturated fats rather than toward it.

THE LOW-FAT, HIGH-SUGAR DIET GIVES US GUM DISEASE AND DIABETES

If the lipid–heart hypothesis has one serious, tragic failure, it's that the type 2 diabetes epidemic has arisen during its tenure. I see the signs of blood sugar dysfunction in red, bleeding, and infected gums all the time. People with diabetes are at a higher risk of periodontal (gum) disease.[26] If diabetes is undiagnosed or left to worsen, it can make gum disease even worse, leading to acute infections and, in severe cases, tooth loss.

Up until the 1970s, type 2 diabetes affected less than 2 percent of the U.S. population. But since that time, the numbers have ballooned, and today 29 million Americans—just under 10 percent of the population—suffers from type 2 diabetes.[27]

There was a dramatic spike in diabetes during the mid-1990s, about the second decade of when the low-fat diet was popular. On a personal note, I remember my mother replacing our butter with margarine, our salad dressings with their low-fat, high-sugar alternatives, and our milk with nonfat powdered milk around that time. The milk tasted like water and the margarine tasted like nothing, but she said it was healthier, so we accepted it. There's no doubt that millions of families around the globe made similar unfortunate changes. And that those changes further fueled the rise of type 2 diabetes.

The key lies with insulin. When glucose levels rise to a certain point, the pancreas releases insulin, which helps the body use glucose for energy or store it as fat. The more glucose we ingest, the more insulin we have to make, and the more fat our body stores.

Weight gain and metabolic syndrome* are not a calorie issue; they're a hormone issue. When we eat sugar, the glucose in it spikes our blood sugar, which tells our body to release insulin and store fat.[28] At the same time, fructose goes to our liver and has to be converted into fat, causing inflammation and also a resistance to insulin.[29]

In nature, glucose and fructose—simple sugars—are always packaged with complex carbs, or fiber, like the skin of an apple or the crunchy outside of a string bean. These additions make it easier for our bodies to process the simple sugars.

But the low-fat, high-sugar foods that families like mine turned to have added simple sugars *without* the counterbalancing complex carbs or fiber. Simple sugars now dominate everything from soft drinks to cereals to baked goods to countless other foods we never think twice about.

The more we consume these foods, the more our bodies became resistant to insulin. Many people's bodies get to the point

---

* The Mayo Clinic defines metabolic syndrome as "a cluster of conditions—increased blood pressure, high blood sugar, excess body fat around the waist, and abnormal cholesterol or triglyceride levels—that occur together, increasing your risk of heart disease, stroke and diabetes."

where they don't respond to insulin at all, they can't process the sugar intake from the diet, and their blood sugar becomes dangerously high. That's type 2 diabetes.

High blood sugar can damage the outer structure of HDLs, making them less recognizable to other cells,[30] and can also damage LDLs,[31] further contributing to the risk of heart disease.[32] As a final insult, the incidence of nonalcoholic fatty liver disease is on a sharp rise, due to our livers trying to cope with fructose.[33] Fructose's metabolic impact on our livers is similar to the impact of chronic alcoholism.[34]

In other words, in our effort to stay on a low-fat diet to protect ourselves from heart disease, we end up eating more sugar. This can mess up the way we process fat and put us at risk of heart disease after all—in addition to making us more vulnerable to tooth decay, gum disease, fatty liver, and diabetes. Talk about the cure being worse than the disease!

Today many doctors are working to reverse these mistaken trends. Just like gum disease and diabetes, fatty liver (and other organs) and even insulin resistance is spreading to younger and younger children. Robert Lustig, a pediatric physician and author of the book *Fat Chance*, has shown that simply removing fructose from children's diets can dramatically reduce their markers for type 2 diabetes and liver fat in the span of 10 days.[35] And now doctors who long recommended the low-fat diet for healthy hearts are recommending higher-fat diets.

NATURE KNOWS WHAT IT'S DOING

One of the overarching lessons I hope you take from this book is that, as products of nature, our bodies were designed to take in foods as they exist *in nature*. When we cut out whole categories of nutrients, and when we refine and process food, we pay a certain price.

Though it was started with good intentions, the low-fat movement ignored this important rule. The result was generations of kids that grew up on a diet high in processed, refined sugar, white flour, and seed oils.

When kids eat a low-fat diet that's high in simple carbohydrates like sugar, they get tooth decay. They don't get the nutrients and minerals that the body needs to create strong, healthy teeth and bones. And they put themselves at risk of the metabolic chaos of obesity, heart disease, and type 2 diabetes.

Today we simply do not consume foods that provide the fat-soluble vitamins and other nutrients we need to fix these wrongs. In order to correct course, we need to remove the stigma associated with fat and move on from the low-fat movement. The next chapters will help you do that yourself.

PART III

DENTAL NUTRITION— HOW TO EAT FOR A HEALTHY MOUTH, BODY, AND MIND

CHAPTER 9

EATING TO MAKE YOUR DENTAL CHECKUP A BREEZE

To develop the Dental Diet, I looked for foods that would satisfy four main objectives, based on the principles we've talked about throughout this book. Let's call them the principles of good dental nutrition.

THE PRINCIPLES OF GOOD DENTAL NUTRITION

1. Keep the jaw, face, and airways healthy and strong.
2. Give the mouth the nutrients it needs (with a focus on calcium balance and the fat-soluble vitamins).
3. Keep the microbiome balanced and diverse.
4. Eat foods with healthy epigenetic messages.

Now let's talk about how the Dental Diet specifically satisfies each of these principles.

1. KEEP THE JAW, FACE, AND AIRWAYS HEALTHY AND STRONG.

Healthy chewing

The jaw is a biomechanical joint that requires stimulation to develop properly and stay healthy and strong. The muscles, joints, and bones in the face form the support structure for your airways, so exercising your jaw also helps keep your airways healthy.

We're meant to get our jaw exercise from chewing, one of the few ways to keep it strong and functioning properly. (There aren't a lot of exercise routines or machines at the gym designed for the mouth and jaw!) When we eat processed, mushy, or highly refined foods, we deny our jaw this exercise. The Dental Diet prioritizes hard, fibrous foods that require chewing, thereby developing the jaw throughout your adult life. These foods include:

- Whole raw vegetables
- Whole nuts and seeds
- Meat on the bone
- Chewy dried or cured meats

Healthy breathing

Every time you breathe, you exert an expanding force on your maxilla, or upper jaw. If you breathe improperly (usually through your mouth), your teeth can drift or become crooked, your facial muscles don't work as they should, and you slowly starve your body of the number one nutrient it needs: oxygen. Breathing through your nose is essential for your health.

Proper nasal breathing requires the proper posture of your tongue sitting at the roof of your mouth with the tip just behind your front teeth, which trains the muscles of the neck and throat to support your airways. It also exerts forces that expand and maintain your palate (which houses your upper teeth and nasal airways). But it also mixes the air you breathe with nitrous oxide, which increases the blood flow to your blood vessels and helps your body to absorb more oxygen.

Breathing for good digestion

Breathing impacts your digestion, too.

You might be familiar with the fight-or-flight response. It's your body's built-in survival system, designed to respond to life-threatening situations. If you encounter a tiger in nature, you are designed to either fight or take flight. Either way, your body turns on the sympathetic nervous system. It increases your heart rate, your breathing, and the flow of blood to your limbs. It directs blood away from organs and the digestive system.

The sympathetic nervous system is balanced by the parasympathetic nervous system. It slows your heart rate and stimulates the organs in your digestive tract.

Breathing is one of the body's ways to control the balance of these systems. Fast, shallow breathing, focusing on the inhale turns on the sympathetic nervous system; slow, deep breathing, focusing on the exhale, activates the parasympathetic nervous system.

Tip: Before every meal, take five deep, slow breaths through your nose. Breathe in for 3 seconds and breathe out for 4 to 5 seconds. This will help to switch on your parasympathetic nervous system, and you'll absorb nutrients from food more effectively.

2. GIVE THE MOUTH THE NUTRIENTS IT NEEDS.

Fat-soluble vitamins

In addition to helping the body use and distribute calcium, each fat-soluble vitamin plays several important roles in the body and is found in specific foods in nature.

Vitamin D

Vitamin D is absolutely fundamental to our health. To start, our digestive system needs it to absorb calcium from the food we eat—the calcium that our body uses to grow and strengthen our teeth and bones. Vitamin D is vital to countless other processes and organs, such as our metabolism, immune system, and even our brain function.

Our bodies are designed to synthesize vitamin D from the sun, so it's ideal to get at least half an hour of sunlight during the middle hours of the day. This is when sunlight contains UVB rays, which trigger our skin to convert a prohormone (a sort of inactivated hormone) into vitamin D.

If you work indoors or you have health problems preventing you from getting outside, you may not be synthesizing enough vitamin D from sunlight. If you live in a place that's higher than 37 degrees north latitude or lower than 37 degrees south, you probably won't be able to get enough ultraviolet rays for your body to convert to vitamin D, no matter what you do. Since our modern environment isn't the most conducive to receiving the necessary amount of vitamin D, most of us should try to obtain vitamin D from our diet.

The best sources of vitamin D are animal products, like fatty fish, liver, cheese, and egg yolks. In animals, vitamin D comes in a form that our bodies can use more efficiently. The form of D that comes in plants (vitamin D2) is harder for our bodies to process.

Vitamin A

Vitamin A is important for your body to grow and repair itself. It supports a healthy immune system and also good eyesight. You may recognize that carrots are a good source of vitamin A. Like vitamin D, vitamin A that comes from plants needs to be converted into its active form to be used in the human body. Carotenoids—pigments that help turn plants red, yellow, and orange—are often confused with vitamin A. But our bodies actually have to convert them into retinol, the active form of vitamin A, before they can use them.

There are many things that help the body to convert vitamin A. For instance, cooking vegetables and fruits in fat helps. But as a rule, plant foods are a less potent source of vitamin A than animal foods.

I recommend that nearly all of my patients take cod-liver oil after the biggest meal of the day. It's a great source of vitamins D, A, and various essential fatty acids. Cod liver wraps them all up in one neat, metabolically available package.

Make sure to read directions written on packages for food sources of vitamin A for the recommended daily limit. If you're unsure about your needs, consult your physician.

Vitamin K2

Vitamin K2 is crucial for your bone and teeth health. It's also important in making sure calcium stays out of your blood vessels.

When animals consume vitamin K1, which is found in grass and green, leafy vegetables, their digestive system converts it into K2. This is another reason that grass-fed animals produce healthier meat than grain-fed animals.

Eggs from pasture-raised chickens and butter from grass-fed cows are good sources of MK-4 vitamin K2. So are organ meats, shellfish, and emu oil.

MK-7 vitamin K2 is formed through the fermentation of bacteria, so fermented foods can be a good source of this type of vitamin K2. These foods include natto, sauerkraut, and cheeses like Gouda and brie.

If you take warfarin, consult with a physician about your vitamin K intake. Dietary vitamin K can interfere with warfarin activity in the body.

3. KEEP THE MICROBIOME BALANCED AND DIVERSE.

To a large degree, your overall health depends on the health of the microbiome in your mouth and gut. It needs a balance of "good" slow-metabolizing bacteria and "bad" fast-metabolizing bacteria.

When you sit down to eat a meal, be aware that you're now feeding the trillions of microbes inside of you. These thriving organisms depend on the food you put in your mouth for their survival, so the fate of that balance is in your hands (or at least on your fork).

To keep everyone happy, you need to consume a balance of foods that contains *probiotics* and *prebiotics*.

Probiotics

If there's anything about food that traditional societies had a better appreciation of than we do, it was the relationship between the microbes in their food and the microbes in their bodies.

Traditional societies had to preserve their foods, and fermentation was an effective way of doing it. These fermented foods were carefully cultured with live microbes that both replenished and reinvigorated the good bacteria in the gut.

Every meal should both feed and replenish microbes in order to keep them thriving and diverse, which keeps the harmful ones from taking over. It sounds strange, but when you eat, you should ask yourself, "Am I eating microbes in this meal?"

Prebiotics (fiber)

The word *prebiotics* refers to any food ingredient that feeds the bacteria in our gut. In a testament to how important prebiotics are, human breast milk is full of prebiotic factors that are crucial in establishing a baby's gut flora and digesting the milk itself.

Prebiotics are mainly found in fiber. Broadly, fiber is complex carbohydrates that our digestive system doesn't break down itself but uses to feed the microbes that live within our mouth and digestive system. Only plant foods contain fiber.

Science generally divides dietary fiber into two categories: soluble and insoluble. Soluble fiber dissolves in water, while insoluble fiber does not. In the body, insoluble fiber is generally recognized as giving our stool "bulk." But it's more likely that its real role is feeding many different types of microbes in the digestive system that we haven't yet characterized.

The human microbiome is hugely diverse, and we're really just beginning to learn about the impact that different types of fiber have on it. But one thing is already clear: To have a healthy microbiome, you need to eat a lot of fiber, and most people certainly don't eat enough.

4. EAT FOOD WITH HEALTHY EPIGENETIC MESSAGES.

Each of your genes can be expressed in a staggering number of ways. Epigenetic messages determine how they're expressed. The healthier those messages are, the healthier your cells, organs, and ultimately your genes will be.

The food you eat contains not just nutrients that you absorb, but the collective epigenetic messages that eventually shape your gut bacteria, immune system, metabolism, and hormones as well. As you digest food, a flood of nutrients and bacteria move through your body; they interact with each other and trigger epigenetic messages that eventually flow down to your genes.

At the simplest level, the presence of a certain nutrient will methylate your DNA, or turn certain genes on, while the absence of another nutrient will switch certain genes off. These messages affect how our bodies operate. Methylation or lack of it may result in long-term weight gain, for instance, or increase the insulin resistance of a cell, or affect certain neurological functions.

The fat-soluble vitamins are central to gene regulation, and their presence is one of the most powerful and positive epigenetic messages we can send to our bodies. But nutrients alone don't influence our epigenetic messages.

The foods we eat have their own microbiomes, and their bacterial balance is tied up in an intimate lattice with their own genes. This epigenetic fingerprint is shaped by how the food is raised (if it's an animal) or grown (if it's a plant). When we eat food, its epigenetic fingerprint speaks to our own microbiome, which responds to the messages it holds, and eventually relays messages to our own genes. It's an intimate and complex conversation.

Scientists are only just beginning to understand the relationship between microbes and genes. A recent study has demonstrated that short-chain fatty acids have the ability to directly alter DNA by way of epigenetic messaging.[1] You'll remember that these fatty acids are produced by bacteria in the stomach when we eat fermentable fibers, establishing a direct relationship between food, microbes, and your genes.

Your health, in part, is a response to all those messages. One wrong message might result in a hole in your tooth or lead to an autoimmune disease. Chronic diseases are a result of eating foods that ruin our epigenetic fingerprint. It's important to remember that every meal is an opportunity to make sure your microbiome and your genes are getting the right epigenetic messages from your food.

Food sourcing

If an animal doesn't see sunlight, doesn't graze on grass, or is dosed with antibiotics, then its body composition changes. This means that the epigenetic messages in its cells change, too—and probably not for the better.

Cows raised on grain and not grass have their fatty acid profile changed from a ratio that's higher in omega-3 (anti-inflammatory) fatty acids to one that's higher in omega-6s (inflammatory). Without grass and sunlight, their milk doesn't contain the fat-soluble vitamins D, A, and K2 that naturally occur in their own digestive system, and they aren't converting sunlight to vitamin D.

It's important to know where your food lived its life. You can directly control the epigenetic messages that your food sends to your genes by buying fresh, locally grown produce from farmers who understand how nature nurtures health.

Animal products should be sourced from:

- Pasture-raised animals and free-range livestock
- Seafood caught in natural waters. (Like their land-based counterparts, wild-caught fish have fatty acid profiles that are different from those of farmed and grain-fed fish.)
- Crops that haven't been sprayed with pesticides and antibiotics, which shift the microbiome of their soil as well as that of their own genes.

Nature's perfect food?

I'm a big believer that our bodies are uniquely designed to make use of the resources and nutrients that nature gives us. Our bodies are constantly telling us, reminding us, and giving us clues about what's good for us. They teach us about our own health. We just have to listen.

As we've learned, our mouth is a great example of this. If there is one food that shows us how to eat for dental health, it's breast milk. Breast milk shows us which nutrients a growing baby needs to develop a healthy body and mouth. From there, we can extrapolate what we need for a healthy body and mouth throughout our lives. What's more, the act of breastfeeding shows us how to develop and maintain strong jaws and airways.

In fact, breast milk and breast-feeding helped me model the Dental Diet. Here's how they satisfy the principles of good dental (and overall) nutrition that I listed above:

1. **Keep the jaw, face, and airways healthy and strong.**

    Breast-feeding gives babies facial exercise at the earliest stage of life. Breast-feeding is trigged by the rooting reflex, which engages five cranial nerves. Babies learn to use their tongue muscles, which helps support their airways. The tongue posture helps develop their autonomic nervous system, in particular the vagus nerve, which is crucial for digestive balance in the body.[2]

    In order to extract milk from the breast, babies learn to use their tongue to push the mother's nipple against their palate, which helps to develop their upper jaw and prevent crooked teeth.[3] Breast-feeding also teaches babies to breathe through their nose. This is extra important since nasal breathing mixes the air we take in with nitrous oxide, which helps our body absorb more oxygen.

2. **Give the mouth the nutrients it needs (with a focus on calcium and the fat-soluble vitamins).**

    Breast milk is exquisitely designed to give a baby's growing body the nutrients it needs. The mother's body makes careful calculations of how much of the nutrients she can spare. When there's a sufficient amount of a certain nutrient, it gets passed to the baby through the breast milk. When there isn't a sufficient amount, the baby may suffer from the deficiency as well.

    For instance, if a woman with a vitamin D deficiency breast-feeds her baby, there's a good chance the baby will have a vitamin D shortage as well.[4] This is likely also the case for vitamins A and K2. Many traditional societies would make sure that a mother's prenatal diet had plenty of fat-soluble, vitamin-rich foods. This would ensure that a mother had plenty of stores for both herself and her child.

3. **Keep the microbiome balanced and diverse.**

   Breast milk does an excellent job of establishing the microbiome of the baby. Breast milk was long thought to be sterile, but recently we've learned that it transports bacteria from a mother's gut to her child's oral and then gut microbiome. It's full of both prebiotic factors and live microbes that serve as the starter pack for the newborn's developing digestive and immune systems.[5]

4. **Eat food with healthy epigenetic messages.**

   The composition of breast milk varies during the lactation period, but it's not the macronutrient composition of fats, carbohydrates, and proteins that changes. Instead, the bioactive components, including immunological factors and fatty acids that send epigenetic messages, evolve. This suggests that a mother's body is sending different environmental— and epigenetic—growth signals to the child.[6]

THE SUPPORT NUTRIENTS

You'll notice that there are plenty of vitamins and minerals not mentioned above (vitamins B and C, for example). We could spend an entire book or series of books going over every nutrient we need and what it does in the body. But the Dental Diet focuses on the foods that supply the most crucial and select set of key nutrients. The fat-soluble vitamins require a very particular sourcing and preparation of foods in order for us to get enough in our diet. When we design a diet around them, nature delivers the other nutrients with them.

In addition to vitamins D, A, and K2, there are a handful of support nutrients that broadly round out the fat-soluble system.

Calcium

One of the most important jobs your body has is to maintain its hard skeletal structures. Odontoblasts need calcium to build and maintain your teeth, and osteoblasts need it to build your bones.

The trouble with calcium is that if it builds up in the wrong places, it can cause anything from tooth decay to heart disease. To control the flow of calcium and fully utilize it, your body needs fat-soluble vitamins. The condition of your teeth is a good sign of whether it's getting them. In this way, it's a good sign of your overall health.

One of the biggest misconceptions about calcium is that, if someone's bones become weak (as in osteoporosis), they need *more* calcium. As we've discussed, it's more likely that they have enough calcium already but don't have enough of the fat-soluble vitamins that let their bodies *make use of it.*

In some cases, calcium supplements (especially in the form of calcium carbonate) have been found to have little impact on bone density and may even be harmful to our health. It's best to consume calcium in its biologically absorbable forms, including dairy, green vegetables (especially dark, leafy greens), almonds, whole fish, and soups with meat cooked on the bone.

Fat and cholesterol

Fats aren't water-soluble, so our digestive system has very specific mechanisms to move it around the body. And these mechanisms depend on fat itself. To get fat-soluble vitamins and many other crucial nutrients where they need to go, and for our cells to absorb them, we need to *eat* certain fats.

For the most part, your small intestine breaks down fats. Your liver produces bile, which combines with a complex mix of enzymes from the pancreas, to break down fats and turn them into droplets that your small intestine can absorb. The catch is that the main ingredient of bile is cholesterol, so cholesterol itself plays a key role in how we process fats. Your body is capable of producing its own cholesterol, but it also needs dietary sources of cholesterol.

Once they're absorbed in the small intestine, the fats get packaged into the all-important lipoproteins that deliver them, along with the fat-soluble vitamins and other nutrients, all over the body. Needless to say, this is a complex process in which many different compounds play key roles; you can't afford to leave any of them out. Your body needs the full range of dietary fats (50 percent of which should be saturated fats) to fully absorb the fat-soluble vitamins and other fat-soluble nutrients.

In order for this to happen, your body needs all kinds of fats. These include:

- *Saturated*—meats, tallow, lard, butter, cheese
- *Monounsaturated*—olive oil, peanuts, almonds, avocados
- *Polyunsaturated*—fish, walnuts, flaxseed
- *Cholesterol*—liver, fish, eggs, butter

Magnesium

You may remember the high school experiment where you burn magnesium to create a bright white light. That's a good shorthand view of what magnesium does in the body; it's the catalyst for more than 300 specific chemical reactions, including every reaction that depends on adenosine triphosphate, or ATP, the "universal energy currency of our cells,"[7] something like a cellular battery.

Magnesium is crucial for your cells, as it activates the enzyme that makes copies of DNA and the enzyme that makes RNA, which is responsible for relaying the instructions in our genes to our cells. Our cells then use these instructions to make every protein in our body, a process also known as gene expression. Vitamins A and D carry out most of their jobs in the process of gene expression, so they, too, rely directly on magnesium to function properly. Magnesium also plays a crucial role in the receptors and proteins that vitamins A and D interact with.

The interaction between magnesium, vitamin D, and calcium is a good example of magnesium's importance. Our body converts vitamin D to the active compound calcitriol, which helps regulate gene expression and stimulates the absorption of calcium. But this process relies on magnesium. So people who are deficient in magnesium have low blood levels of both calcitriol and calcium, but giving them vitamin D supplements doesn't necessarily restore their calcium levels to normal.[8] Their body needs sufficient amounts of magnesium to make vitamin D work the way it's supposed to. Magnesium also supports the cellular pumps that keep most calcium out of our soft tissue and make it available for our bones and teeth.

Foods rich in magnesium include spinach, pumpkin seeds, avocado, black beans, yogurt, dark chocolate, and bananas.

Zinc

Zinc helps maintain the structural integrity of the proteins in our bodies, and alongside magnesium, it helps regulate gene expression.[9] Zinc also plays a key role in how our bodies process vitamin A.[10] Vitamin A helps our intestines absorb zinc, and in turn, zinc supports the transport of vitamin A and the other fat-soluble vitamins across the intestinal wall.

Zinc is also an essential structural component of many vitamin A–related proteins, including the main protein that transports vitamin A through the blood and the proteins that let vitamin A influence gene expression.

Foods rich in zinc include beef, lamb, chicken, pumpkin seeds, spinach, mushrooms, cashews, and chickpeas.

Gelatin

Collagen is one of the most crucial structural building blocks of our skin, joints, gums, and all of our other connective tissues. Our bodies make collagen out of the amino acids glycine and proline. (Glycine is also a likely factor in normal growth and development in the way it helps to release human growth hormone.[11])

Sometimes the body is unable to repair its own connective tissues. For example, in people with gum disease, chronic inflammatory processes lead to the breakdown of these tissues. The human body can synthesize glycine and proline on its own, but their vast roles mean we should aim to get more through the food we eat to replenish its supplies.

Dietary collagen is found in its natural state mainly in animal connective tissue. That's why broths and soups with meat cooked on the bone—joints and cartilage and all—are important to our health. They're among the few dietary sources of collagen, which, when cooked, turns to gelatin. Broths and meat stocks also contain calcium, magnesium, and other trace minerals released from joints. Traditional societies have long made broths or meat stocks fundamental parts of their diets, likely for this reason.

The bottom line is that a healthy diet *necessarily* includes animal products with gelatin-rich skin, bone marrow, collagenous joints, and slow-cooked stocks and broths.

THE PROGRAM

For thousands of years, humans didn't need to consider "dietary recommendations" or adjust their meals to monthly snap diets. Eating was simple. They ate food as they found it in the environment.

Today we have the very fortunate problem of being surrounded by food, but that means we need to be able to discern which foods will promote our health and which ones won't.

The mouth is a great model for showing us which foods are good for us. What's good for dental health is good for overall health. That's why we've established the four dietary goals above.

In order to work toward these goals, we have to identify and remove the modern foods that pull us away from them and cause illness. We also need to learn to identify the foods that provide us with vital, fat-soluble vitamins. Last, we need to incorporate foods that enhance our microbiome, an organ and biological entity in its own right. The following program will show you how to put this all into action.

STEP 1: ELIMINATE

The first step is to identify and remove the harmful foods and ingredients that regularly reach your plate. Your overall strategy should be to remove all packaged and refined foods from your diet and to monitor the meals you have when you eat out, making sure they're cooked in the proper ways with the proper ingredients.

At a glance

- Refined vegetable oils: NONE
- White flour: NONE.
- Sugar: Maximum added sugar intake per week: 6 teaspoons for women, 9 teaspoons for men (1 teaspoon = 4.2 grams)

Guidelines

1. **Remove vegetable oils**

    The bad news is that removing refined vegetable oils from your diet can be difficult because they're everywhere. They're used to prepare nearly all packaged foods, all the food we can get in supermarkets, and all the food we can order in restaurants.

    The good news is that vegetable oils don't add any flavor to food; if anything, they can dull flavor. So eliminating them, and eating more natural fat, often makes foods taste better and feels more satisfying.

    Avoid the following vegetable oils:
    Canola/rapeseed oil, soybean oil, corn oil, sunflower oil, safflower oil, and peanut oil.

    Replace them with:
    Coconut oil; animal fats including lard, tallow, butter, and ghee; avocado oil; or olive oil.

2. Remove white flour

This can be a challenge if you're used to eating bread, pasta, or white rice. And yes, I realize that covers just about all of us. But it's worth it. Removing white flour can have an amazing effect on your health.

It's okay to substitute whole-grain alternatives to white flour, but you should stick to no more than two to three servings of even whole grains per week. In fact, I recommend eliminating *all* grains from your diet for at least two weeks to let your body feel what it's like to live without them. That will also give you an objective baseline to measure against if you eat them again.

I enjoy eating whole grains occasionally, but I find that I feel better overall if I keep it at two to three times per week. Whole grains include brown rice, barley, oats, millet, spelt, and quinoa.

Remove:
Flour, rice, pasta, breads, crackers, and packaged cereals

Replace with:
Carrots, beans, lentils, and chickpeas

3. Remove sugar

For many of us, sugar has an addictive effect on our body. Eliminating it is probably the biggest challenge in the Dental Diet. Even when you replace sugar with the right foods, your body almost always goes through some kind of withdrawal period. My patients have experienced headaches, cloudiness, fatigue, body aches, jitters, trouble sleeping, and even flulike symptoms. These effects don't usually persist for more than five days, but in rare cases they can last longer.

I recommend cutting out all sugar from your diet for at least two weeks, which includes eliminating fruit. I find that my patients seem to escape the clutches of sugar addiction only if they eliminate it altogether for at least two weeks. This resets your taste buds and your hunger cycle and allows your body to recognize and crave foods that are actually good for you.

Am I quitting sugar for life?

I'm not saying you have to quit sugar for life. But I do think that once you give your body the time it needs to get *over* sugar, you won't feel nearly as attached to it, anyway. You'll find that adding sugar to your coffee or tea or downing that sugar-packed pastry isn't as appealing as it once was.

You won't have any more afternoon or late-night sugar cravings because your body will understand that it doesn't need sugar at all. You'll also lose weight. And of course, tooth decay will be much less of a worry.

Remove:
Packaged food that has more than 5 to 6 grams of sugar per 100 grams.

Avoid:

- Bottled, flavored drinks, including sports drinks. Drink water instead.
- Fruit juices—these contain all of the sugar but none of the healthy fiber of fruits.
- Cereals—including the "healthy" brands. Cereals are a minefield of white flour and sugar. It's important to keep away from anything that resembles a packaged cereal you could buy at the supermarket.
- Salad dressings
- Sauces
- Canned foods

Other sources of sugar to watch

Dairy

Dairy contains lactose, which is a sugar that breaks down into galactose and glucose. Full-fat dairy products naturally contain, on average, about 4.7 grams of lactose, or sugar. Any additional sugar is added sugar. If you can tolerate it, it's fine to consume lactose, and you don't need to add it to your daily sugar tally since your body doesn't turn it into fructose.

Fruit

Generally, I recommend eating no more than two to three pieces of fruit per day. And in weeks 2 and 3 of the program, we completely cut fruit from the diet, in order to cut out sugar entirely. Remember to minimize your consumption of fruit juices, which are concentrated doses of simple sugars.

Alcohol

Drink alcohol in moderation. I don't recommend cutting out alcohol entirely because fermented drinks like beer and wine have very little fructose. The biggest sugar traps with alcohol are mixers and dessert wines. Avoid them.

Artificial sweeteners and "natural" sweeteners

Generally, it's better to avoid artificial and even natural sweeteners, like stevia, because they don't allow your palate to appreciate flavors in nutrient-dense foods that provide fat-soluble vitamins. Changing your palate is the key to reducing your sugar intake in the long term, so I recommend you stay away from anything sweet that would interfere with that process.

STEP 2: BUILD

One of the main lessons I'd like you to take away from *The Dental Diet* is that you shouldn't focus on eating the right *amount* of food; you should focus on eating the right *kinds* of food that are rich in the nutrients your body needs most. Fat-soluble vitamins feed and maintain our mineral balance, our digestive and immune systems, and many other systems in our bodies.

Every meal should contain sources of the fat-soluble vitamins A, D, and K2, as well as the support elements that work alongside them in the body, including magnesium, zinc, and dietary fat.

Foods rich in vitamins, A, D, and K2

- Whole, full-fat animal products, including the skin: beef, chicken, lamb, and duck
- Organ meats
- Whole fish and shellfish
- Milk, butter, yogurt, and cheese
- Eggs
- Natto
- Colorful vegetables and salads cooked or dressed in fat

Support elements

- Magnesium—Pumpkin seeds, leafy greens, dark chocolate (no added sugar)
- Zinc—Kidney beans, flaxseed, shrimp
- Calcium—Dairy, leafy greens, soups and broths
- Dietary fat—Coconut oil, olive oil, lard, tallow
- Gelatin—Skin, joints, bones

STEP 3: BALANCE

Fiber—lots of it

Cutting out refined simple carbohydrates will effectively create microbial chaos in your body, and you will have to rebalance the microbial populations in your mouth and gut. To do this, you need a balance of *probiotics* to deliver and replenish the "good" flora in your microbiomes and *prebiotics* to feed those benevolent bacteria.

Eating more vegetables is a simple and healthy way to do this. Basing every meal on a good foundation of vegetables helps deliver the full range of soluble and insoluble fibers your microbes need to function properly.

Probiotics

It's important to add probiotics—along with prebiotics—to your diet to balance your microbiome. There's already a huge trend of taking probiotics, often in the form of supplements. However, I always try to impress upon my patients that the best source of beneficial microbes is food itself.

The live microbes that live in cultured food both replenish and reinvigorate the good bacteria in your gut. Every meal should be carefully crafted to keep the "good" microbes thriving and to keep the harmful ones from taking over.

Probiotics are found in fermented foods. To keep your microbiome healthy, you should aim to have two to three doses of fermented foods per day. That amounts to just one spoonful of sauerkraut per meal. Other sources of probiotics include pickled vegetables, kombucha, kimchi, active cultured yogurt, cheese, butter, kefir, miso, ciders, and vinegars.

Prebiotics (fermentable fibers)

The different types of fiber are classified as soluble and insoluble, but a more useful classification might be fermentable and nonfermentable. Prebiotics are the soluble fibers that specific microbes consume, via fermentation in the colon, to produce short-chain fatty acids. While these fibers are specifically referred to as prebiotics, the term really refers only to the fibers that we *know* bacteria can convert to short-chain fatty acids. We have identified two of them, inulin and fructo-oligosaccharide, and it's important to eat *plenty* of the foods that contain them. These foods include artichokes, asparagus, onions, leeks, bananas, chives, chicory root, dandelion greens, and garlic.

There are many types of fibers, but the truth is we don't fully know how our bodies process all of them. Still, many of them are likely beneficial to our microbiome, and that's why we should consume other types of fibers in a range of vegetables, legumes, nuts, and seeds. While we should specifically focus on prebiotic fibers, eating a wide variety of plant foods is important. As in all things, diversity is key.

WAKING UP TO THE RIGHT FOODS

As the saying goes: Give a man a fish, and feed him for a day; teach a man to fish, and feed him for life. The main goal of the Dental Diet isn't to get you to remove certain foods from your diet. The main goal is to get you to *see* food differently, which will help you eat healthily for life.

By now you should feel armed with a sharp, questioning, and logical lens for looking at food. Yes, there are harmful foods we need to stay away from. But more important, we need to respect the foods that our bodies really need, and respect the more traditional, natural ways of preparing those foods.

In the next chapter, we'll start to look at the specific food groups—and foods—that fit the Dental Diet.

CHAPTER 10

THE DENTAL DIET MODEL AND FOOD PYRAMID

As mentioned, the Dental Diet is based on four principles of dental nutrition, which in turn are based on traditional diets and nutrient-rich foods:

1. Keep the jaw, face, and airways healthy and strong.
2. Give the mouth the nutrients it needs.
3. Keep the microbiome balanced and diverse.
4. Eat food with healthy epigenetic messages.

These principles helped me form the Dental Diet food pyramid. The pyramid outlines a guide to the relative proportions of each food we need for good dental health. It doesn't talk about "servings" in terms of amount—in the Dental Diet, you don't need to weigh or measure your food. You eat until you're satisfied!

Before we get to it, let's look at a food pyramid you're already familiar with. It's the food pyramid that dominated U.S. dietary recommendations in the 1990s and largely persists in standard recommendations to this day. I want to go over it before show-ing you the Dental Diet pyramid because, whether you're con-scious of it or not, it probably determines how you look at food.

The pyramid outlined how many servings of food we should have every day from each major food group. Generally speak-ing, the U.S. government designed it to be consistent with the concerns and principles behind the low-fat craze of the 1970s, '80s, and '90s. It's easy to see that.

The old pyramid implied that fat was the enemy of a healthy diet. The foods lowest in fat were lower on the pyramid, meaning you should eat more of them, and foods higher in fat (like dairy, meat, and oils) were higher up where the pyramid narrowed, meaning you should eat less of them.

The pyramid exhibited little concern for simple sugars, white flour, polyunsaturated vegetable oils, and refined, processed foods. In fact, it endorsed these foods in no uncertain terms since bread, cereal, rice, and pasta formed its very base.

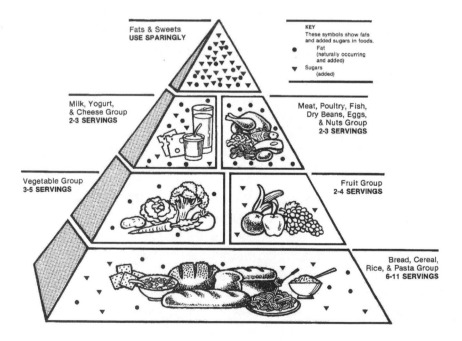

Fig. 23. The original USDA food pyramid guideline for healthy eating

The pyramid didn't account for many of the principles of healthy eating that our ancestors had developed over thousands of years. It was made without consideration of the microbiome, food sourcing, or the fat-soluble vitamins we need to *make use* of so many nutrients. And needless to say, it didn't address which foods we need to eat for our dental health at all.

THE DENTAL DIET PYRAMID

In developing the Dental Diet, I *started* with the foods we need to eat for healthy mouths and teeth. This naturally led to an emphasis on foods that contain fat-soluble vitamins, the fats that help us process them, and so many other nutrients. It led to specific inclusion of the probiotics and prebiotics we need to balance our microbiomes. And it convinced me to focus on natural foods with natural epigenetic messages.

Eating for a healthy mouth also inspired me to reconnect with the natural foods that traditional societies have long eaten to be healthy. The foods that people ate before the Industrial Revolution weren't based on the foods that were simply *available* but also on those they *needed* for good health. I want this pyramid to reorient your own approach to food in much the same way.

The pyramid doesn't specify the exact amounts of each food to eat, because I don't believe measuring *how much* you eat will in any way help you see *which foods* you should eat. Our world is full of foods our bodies don't recognize, and my main goal for the pyramid is to help you steer your diet away from them and toward the foods that are truly good for you. (An important part of this is recalibrating your view of fats, which our bodies need for energy, for carrying out many cellular functions, and to absorb fat-soluble vitamins.)

If you prioritize the foods you eat according to the tiers in this pyramid, your mouth and body will start functioning as they're actually designed to. They'll begin to fire on all cylinders, so to speak. If you can't eat some of these foods, for whatever reason, that's okay—as long as you make sensible replacements.

Of course, it's not quite enough to eat the *right* foods. It's important that they be sourced and prepared the right way so that by the time they reach your plate, they still have the nutrients you need from them. My model is designed around three principles that protect the nutritional value of the foods you'll eat.

1. **It's best to eat whole foods.**

   Our bodies are designed to process foods as they exist in nature, not as they've been processed, refined, and otherwise manipulated in factories.

2. **It's not just *which* foods you eat, it's how they're prepared.**

   When we prepare foods in different ways, we bring out different nutrients in them. That's why the pyramid divides foods into groups based not only on *type* of food (e.g., vegetables, meats, dairy) but also on how foods are *prepared*. That's why some foods belong to multiple groups. For example, cabbage is in the vegetable group, but it's also in the fermented foods group. Cheese is in the dairy and fermented foods groups.

3. **Sourcing is important, too.**

   As we've discussed, the life of a plant or animal— the conditions in which it grows, the foods it consumes itself—impacts its own microbiome and epigenetics. And when we eat it, those things affect our own health. We want to stick to foods that have been grown or raised in conditions that make sure its microbiome and epigenetics are healthy.

   That means eating animal products from animals raised on grass, whenever possible. It also means eating local, naturally raised fruits and vegetables whenever possible. Getting your food from farmers' markets is a good way to ensure this. It will also let you get to know the people who raise your food, which will deepen your own relationship with what's on your plate.

Let's be realistic . . .

While it's important to eat from the foods in the Dental Diet pyramid as much as you can, I know it won't always be possible. And besides, life is about balance. The Dental Diet model gives you a little wiggle room. If you can stick to the foods in the pyramid 80 percent of the time, or for four out of every five meals, you'll be doing your mouth, teeth, and overall health a big favor. If you limit your intake of modern, processed foods to one out of every five meals at most, your other meals should supply the materials your body needs to overcome a bit of modern food.

The Dental Diet pyramid has four tiers. Generally, you should eat most from the first (bottom) tier. You should eat a little less from the second tier, a bit less from the third, and be particularly mindful of your intake from the top tier.

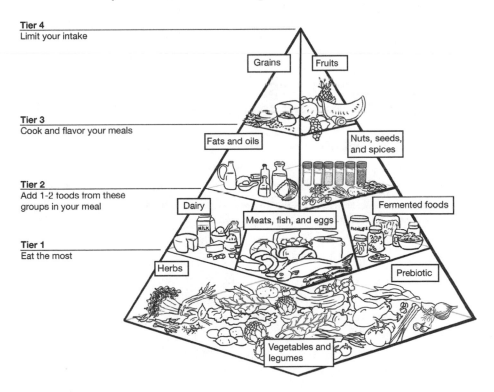

Fig. 24. The Dental Diet Food Pyramid

Tier 1, the base, is composed of plant foods such as vegetables (including those with fermentable prebiotics), legumes, and herbs. These foods should make up the *majority* of every meal.

Tier 2 contains foods that have the crucial nutrients your body needs. You should include foods from one to two of these groups in every meal. The groups in this tier are meats, eggs, fish, dairy (if tolerated), and fermented foods.

Tier 3 includes foods you can cook with or add to your food for flavoring: fats and oils, and nuts, seeds, and spices. These foods make great additions to meals; add them in an amount that makes you *enjoy* your food.

Tier 4 consists of foods you should eat in limited qualities, generally because they contain a lot of simple sugars: grains and fruits.

TIER 1

THE BASE: PLANTS, VEGETABLES, LEGUMES, HERBS, AND PREBIOTICS

A healthy diet is based mainly on plants, or vegetables—we'll use the words interchangeably. Plants are the most abundant food source in nature, and our bodies were designed to take advantage of that fact. That's why vegetables, legumes, herbs, and prebiotics form the base of the Dental Diet pyramid. You should eat two to three foods from this group in every meal. They should be fresh, seasonal, locally sourced, organic vegetables whenever possible.

It's important to eat a *varied* diet of these foods. You can get a lot of different nutrients from plants, but you have to eat a lot of different *parts* of the plants (i.e., leaves, stems, seeds, etc.) to get them.

Vegetables, or plant foods

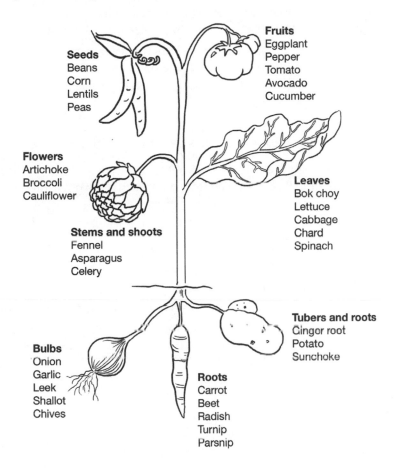

Seeds
Beans
Corn
Lentils
Peas

Fruits
Eggplant
Pepper
Tomato
Avocado
Cucumber

Flowers
Artichoke
Broccoli
Cauliflower

Leaves
Bok choy
Lettuce
Cabbage
Chard
Spinach

Stems and shoots
Fennel
Asparagus
Celery

Tubers and roots
Gingor root
Potato
Sunchoke

Bulbs
Onion
Garlic
Leek
Shallot
Chives

Roots
Carrot
Beet
Radish
Turnip
Parsnip

Fig. 25. Different types of vegetables

Fruits: These are the meaty and nutrient-dense parts of the plant. (We should note that these are "fruits" from a biological standpoint. They shouldn't be confused with the other foods we usually call fruits, like apples, oranges, and grapes, which have large amounts of natural sugars.)

Seeds: The fiber powerhouse of vegetables. They are packed with soluble fiber that slows digestion and helps us absorb nutrients.

Flowers: These give us a great mix of fiber and nutrients.

Stems and shoots: Stems and shoots provide a mix of soluble and insoluble fiber that add bulk to your stools.

Leaves: Leafy greens are rich in phytonutrients that carry many health benefits throughout the body.

Tubers and roots: These are traditionally used as staples due to their starchy, filling nature.

Bulbs: Bulbs are excellent sources of soluble prebiotic fibers that are used by beneficial bacteria in the digestive system.

The more species and colors you have on your plate, the better. You should also make sure to eat a mix of both raw and cooked vegetables.

Legumes

Also known as pulses, legumes are vegetables that usually come in the form of a pod that opens along a seam. Legumes are full of fermentable fibers, proteins, and other nutrients, but they contain some nutrients that may be difficult for some people to digest. Still, many cultures have consumed raw legumes for centuries, if not millennia.

Legumes include:

- Alfalfa
- Beans
- Chickpeas
- Lentils
- Peanuts
- Peas

How to eat legumes

To maximize the digestibility of legumes, it's best to soak them before cooking or eating them.

For kidney-shaped beans: Add water and baking soda in a large pot and soak for 12 to 24 hours before cooking.

For other beans (like black beans): Soak in water and 1 tablespoon of cider vinegar or lemon juice for every cup of dried legumes you use.

Herbs

Herbs are plants that we use for food, flavoring, or medicine. Generally, herbs differ from regular vegetables in that we consume them in small amounts due to their strong fragrance or flavor. The intense taste and aroma of herbs indicates how rich they are in phytochemicals, compounds that are naturally found in plants and have many health benefits. That's why herbs have been used in cooking and medicine throughout human history: They don't just taste great; they're great for our health.

Herbs include:

- Basil
- Dill
- Thyme
- Lavender
- Parsley
- Oregano
- Mint
- Fennel
- Sage

How to eat herbs
Add fresh herbs to any dish, whether cooked or raw, or you can use dried herbs.

Prebiotics

These are the plants that contain soluble fibers that can be fermented by the microbes in our gut. You should be sure to include one prebiotic vegetable in every meal to keep your microbiome balanced.

Prebiotics include:

- Garlic
- Asparagus
- Onion
- Leeks

- Dandelion greens
- Bananas

Tasty ways to add plants to your diet

I realize that to some people, eating a lot of vegetables might seem boring. Don't lose heart: If you have the right ingredients and learn the correct techniques and preparations, you can turn any variety of vegetables into delicious—and still very nourishing—meals.

Pro tip: Always add fat when you're cooking or preparing veggies. Yes, *always*. Whether you add a cold dressing to them, like olive oil or butter, or cook them in a fat like coconut oil, lard, or duck fat, not only will your vegetables taste better, but your body will absorb their nutrients much more efficiently.

Different options for cooking vegetables

To prevent your vegetable-based meals from getting boring, cook them in different ways:

Bake
Cut a mix of vegetables, add a fat like coconut oil, butter, ghee, or lard to them, add salt, herbs, and spices, and bake them in the oven at 375–400 degrees until they turn brown, usually around 20 minutes.

Steam
Cut veggies, put into a steaming pot and leave over boiling water for about 20 minutes. Serve them with salt, pepper, and butter.

Stir-fry
Cut up a variety of different-colored vegetables and throw them in a wok or pan glazed with two to three tablespoons of coconut oil, ghee, or lard. Cook on high heat and stir until brown (usually takes about 10 minutes).

Sauté

This is similar to frying. Use a shallow amount of fat that performs well at high heat, like coconut oil, ghee, or lard, to cook the vegetables all at once, moving them around the pan. The smaller amount of fat prevents "frying" and instead lightly browns the vegetables, preserving the texture of the ingredients.

Grill

For a darker color and a smokier taste, use coconut oil and cook vegetables on the grill.

Raw

Cut your veggies, drizzle them with salt, pepper, olive oil, and vinegar, and have a salad.

Soup or stew

Throw your veggies into a pot of water, bring it to a boil, bring it back to a simmer and let it cook for 30 to 45 minutes.

Ways to base your meals on more vegetables: vegetable-based pasta, rice, and veggie fries. Getting creative with vegetables helps to replace simple carbohydrates, such as white flour–based pasta, white rice, and bread.

Vegetable Pasta

Vegetable pasta is a surprisingly tasty—and much more nutritious— replacement for white flour–based noodles. Use a regular vegetable peeler to carve thin slices of vegetables that resemble spaghetti or other thin pasta. If you want to get a little fancy, buy a spiral slicer to make your vegetable noodles more elegant.

You can use nearly any vegetable to make pasta, but the following veggies will be easiest:

- Zucchini
- Sweet potato
- Carrot

Serve hot: Add some fat and a little spice to the pasta and bake, sauté, steam, or fry until it softens a little. Then serve it with other hot foods.

OR

Serve cold: Use the cold pasta as a base; serve it with other veggies and olive or avocado oil for a colorful, crunchy salad.

PESTO

Pesto is a tasty way to add herbs to any meal. It makes for a delicious pasta sauce, but it's also a great addition to salmon, meat, or salad.

Ingredients

2 to 3 bunches of fresh green herb leaves (basil is the most common, but you can use any herb of your liking)

½ cup pine nuts, or any other nut

½ cup grated Parmesan cheese, or any other hard cheese

1 teaspoon salt

1 to 2 garlic cloves

¼ to ½ cup extra-virgin olive oil

Directions

1. In a blender, combine and blend half of the herbs, nuts, cheese, salt, and garlic. Then blend the full amount. Blend continuously until the mixture turns into a uniform paste. Scrape down the sides of the blender as needed.

2. Add olive oil, in small increments, to moisten the pesto. If you want it to have the consistency of a spread, use less oil. For a sauce, use more.

3. Add salt to taste.

4. You can serve the pesto immediately, or you can save it. Pesto usually stays fresh for several days. If saving, place the pesto in the smallest container possible, thoroughly press and pack it to eliminate air pockets, pour a little olive oil over it, cover it, and store it in the fridge. It should stay fresh for about a week. Pesto can also be frozen for three months.

CAULIFLOWER RICE

Ingredients

Cauliflower

Equipment

Food processor or grater

Directions

1. Preheat oven to 400°F.

2. Remove the leaves from the cauliflower, cut the head into quarters, and remove most of the thick core from each quarter. Then cut each quarter into two or three chunks and toss them in the blender. Blend for 30 seconds or so, until the cauliflower resembles fine rice or couscous. (If you don't have a food processor, you can grate raw cauliflower on the coarse side of a grater. You may be left with a few bigger pieces, which will give the "rice" a chunkier texture.)

3. Bake for 12 minutes or stir-fry it in fat. Add herbs and spices to taste, and you've got a healthy and delicious base for any meal.

VEGETABLE FRIES

Vegetable Fries make a great snack or side dish.

Ingredients

Potato, sweet potato, kale, or cucumber

Directions

1. Preheat oven to 425°F.

2. Cut your vegetable into fingers and place them on a tray with waxed paper.

3. Drizzle them with butter, coconut oil, or olive oil, and sprinkle them with salt. Bake for 10 to 15 minutes or until crisp.

4. Serve the fries warm, or store them for a snack.

TIER 2

MEATS, EGGS, AND FISH; FERMENTED FOODS; AND DAIRY

When possible, we should eat animal products that come from organically raised animals and fish that have been able to roam free and soak up sunlight. We should aim to eat meat from different parts of each animal, including eggs, and an organ meat here and there. (Again, it's all about diversity.)

Group 1—Meats, eggs, and fish

Lean meats

Breast meat, a type of muscle meat, and other lean cuts are the least nutritious part of the animal because they lack fat-soluble vitamins. Lean cuts of meat are great to fill in the gaps in meals, but for the most part, the animal products you eat should be fatty cuts.

Skin and joints

When cooking legs, thighs, and breasts, keep the skin on. Eat as much of the meat as you can, including the skin and cartilaginous parts. Include the larger joint bones in soups and stocks that you cook.

Fish and seafood

Try to eat only ocean-sourced fish and seafood. Farmed fish that aren't raised in their natural environment, like grain-fed cattle, have a different nutrient make-up. Eat all parts of the fish, including the head, skin, and organs. An easy way to make sure you consume all the parts is to choose small fish, which can be eaten whole.

Organs

Otherwise known as offal meats, organs are by far the most nutritious parts of the animal. They're where most of the fat-soluble vitamins are stored.

Note: If you eat organ meats twice a week, you'll get enough of the nutrients they supply. Try to limit your intake to four to five times per week to avoid an excess of vitamin A.

Pro tip: Liver is a one-stop shop for many of the nutrients your body needs. It's a rich source of vitamin C and the fat-soluble vitamins A, D, and K2, and it also provides B6, B12, folate, choline, biotin, magnesium, and zinc. Introducing one slice of liver per week into your diet will go a long way toward helping your body get many of the nutrients and vitamins it needs.

How to prepare organ meats

Organ meats include the liver, kidneys, stomach, intestines, heart, and brain (to name several). There are many ways to cook them and many recipes for tasty organ meat dishes. I've found liver to be the most versatile of the organ meats and the best-liked among people who aren't used to eating them.

Pan fry
Pan fry them like steaks with lard, ghee, or coconut oil. Fry them on low heat, since overcooking results in a dry and rough texture.

Cure
Salt-cured and spiced salumi can be made from the belly of the pig. It can be fried and used in various dishes.

Stir-fry
Dice small amounts of the meat and add them to your vegetable stir-fry.

Mince

Minced organ meats are great for a Bolognese sauce or a casserole. Mix a small amount of organ meats with normal cuts of meat, then season and cook in a sauce for a well-rounded and delicious dish.

Pâté

One of the most flexible and delicious ways to enjoy super-nutritious liver is through pâtés. You can change the taste of the pâté by using different types of liver, like chicken, duck, or lamb liver, and by adding herbs and spices. It's a great way to find out what suits your particular tastes and to get still more variety into your diet.

Ingredients

18 ounces chicken/duck/lamb livers

1 onion, thinly sliced

1 clove garlic

1 bunch any green herb, chopped

3 tablespoons cooking sherry

6 ½ ounces butter, softened

¼ teaspoon sea salt or pink rock salt

¼ teaspoon ground black pepper

⅛ teaspoon ground nutmeg

Directions

1. Put the liver and sliced onion in a saucepan, add 2 to 3 cups of water, and bring to a boil. Then reduce the heat to low and simmer for around 20 minutes, or until the meat is tender.

2. Remove the onion, drain, and discard any portions of liver that have hardened.

3. Place the cooked liver in a blender or food processor and blend until smooth. Add chopped garlic, chopped herbs, sherry, butter, salt, pepper, and nutmeg or other spices. Pulse to blend, stopping periodically to check the consistency.

4. Lightly grease your hands with olive oil or butter and mold the pâté into a mound. Place it in the fridge for 1 hour before serving cold.

Soups and broths

The custom of eating chicken soup when you have a cold did not come from nowhere. Meats, cooked slowly on the bone, have healing powers that traditional cultures have taken advantage of for thousands of years.

In order to extract the nutrient-rich gelatin and other collagenous materials and minerals from meats, you need to make broth out of them by boiling and simmering them in water.

By making your own fresh broth, you can ensure its quality. But if you buy stock, you can check its quality fairly easily. Good stock that has plenty of gelatin will turn to jelly after it's been cooled.

Broths take a long time to cook, but they store well in the fridge or freezer, so you should only have to prepare them every two to four weeks.

CHICKEN BROTH

Equipment

Crockpot or stockpot

Large bowl

Mesh strainer

Ingredients

1 whole chicken or 2 chicken carcasses and 2 feet

2 celery stalks, roughly chopped

2 carrots, roughly chopped

1 onion, roughly chopped

2 to 3 cloves of garlic, roughly chopped

2 tablespoons apple cider vinegar

2 bay leaves, or a bunch of rosemary or any other herb of your choice

Salt and pepper to taste

Directions

1. Place the chicken or chicken carcasses in a crockpot or stockpot and cover with the celery, carrots, onion, and garlic. Add the apple cider vinegar, bay leaves, and the chicken feet, if using.

2. Add enough water to cover all the ingredients.

3. Set the crockpot or stove and stockpot on high until the mixture begins to boil, then turn the temperature to low and leave for 12 to 24 hours.

4. Strain the broth into a pot or large bowl, separating the solids from the liquid.

5. You can store chicken and vegetables separately and eat with broth. However, the chicken and vegetables alone will be devoid of taste and very soft due to the long cooking time.

6. Serve the broth that you will be eating immediately. Chill the remaining broth in the pot in a sinkful of ice-cold water. When cool, store the broth in smaller containers in the fridge for up to 4 to 5 days or in the freezer for 4 to 6 months.

BEEF BROTH

Equipment

Crockpot or stockpot

Mason jars

Roasting pan

Mesh strainer

Ingredients

6 pounds beef bones (marrow bones, knuckle bones, joints, and meaty rib or neck bones, enough to fill approximately ¾ of your pot)

Olive oil

¼ cup vinegar or apple cider vinegar

3 onions, chopped

3 carrots, chopped

3 celery stalks, chopped

Sea salt to taste

2 bay leaves

1 bunch thyme

1 bunch parsley

Directions

1. Preheat oven to 350°F.

2. Place bones in a roasting pan and coat with olive oil (rub with clean hands). Roast in the oven until browned (30 to 60 minutes).

3. Add onions, carrots, and celery stalks to crockpot or stockpot while bones are cooking.

4. Add the browned bones to the pot. Add hot water to roasting pan, and pour liquid into the pot. Stir until browned ingredients are mixed in. Add additional water to cover the bones.

5. Bring to a boil on medium/high heat, and remove the film/foam that rises to the top.

6. Reduce heat to a simmer; cover and cook for at least 12 hours and as long as 72 hours. The longer you cook the stock, the more of the gelatinous materials are released from the joints.

7. For the last half hour, add salt, bay leaves, thyme, and parsley.

8. Strain the broth through a fine-mesh strainer. If you're adding some to a meal, pour it straight into the dish. Chill the broth you will be keeping in an ice bath in the kitchen sink.

9. Store in Mason jars in the fridge for 4 to 5 days, or freeze for 4 to 6 months.

Group 2—Fermented foods

Lacto-fermentation is a way to preserve fresh, raw foods. The process involves adding to the foods a community of beneficial microbes that digest certain parts of it and provide nutrients that promote the growth of balanced microbial colonies. Fermented foods are also a good source of vitamin K2, which is produced by the friendly microbes.

Adding a fermented food like sauerkraut, kombucha, kefir, cultured butter, or cheese to your regular diet will give your microbiome just the support and balance it needs.

Fermented foods are pretty easy to make yourself, and they're much cheaper to make than to buy. But if you do purchase them, make sure that they've been refrigerated, that they haven't been pasteurized, and that no sugar has been added to them.

Here's how you can make three of the simplest fermented foods: kefir, kombucha, and sauerkraut.

MILK KEFIR

Milk kefir is a thick, slightly curdled dairy product made by fermenting milk in a grain culture. It's a great addition to savory meals and a good base for a healthy breakfast. You can also drink it straight from a glass.

Equipment

Glass jar

Towel, paper towel, or paper coffee filter

Rubber band to secure the cover to the jar

Nonmetal stirring utensil

Mesh strainer for removing the kefir grains from the finished kefir

Ingredients

1 to 2 teaspoons active milk kefir grains (you can buy them from a local health store or order them online)

1 quart of cow, goat, or coconut milk (ideally unhomogenized)

Directions

1. Add the kefir grains to milk. Pour into a jar.

2. Cover the jar with cloth secured by a rubber band.

3. Leave the mixture in a warm spot until it is slightly thickened and has a pleasant aroma (generally around 24 hours). This is the when the bacteria break down the simple sugars in the milk. While it's fermenting, the grains will rise to the top. Use the nonmetal spoon to stir and keep as a uniform mixture.

4. After culturing is complete, strain to separate the kefir grains from the finished kefir. The grains can then be used in a new batch of milk.

5. Store the finished kefir in the refrigerator.

KOMBUCHA

One of my favorite ferments is a glass of cool kombucha tea. It has a fantastic mix of microbes. I like recommending it to my patients because, as a tangy, fizzy, cold drink, it's a great substitute for soda. Best of all, cool kombucha tea is simple to make yourself.

Equipment

Stockpot

Clean glass jar with air-tight lid (roughly quart-size) or smaller glass bottles

Ingredients

4 to 5 black tea bags

4 to 5 tablespoons of organic white sugar

2 tablespoons cider vinegar

Commercial kombucha scoby (short for "symbiotic colony of bacteria and yeast"). It's basically a thin, gelatinous slab.

Directions

Note: Make sure to use clean jars and clean, nonmetallic implements. Since you're working with a living culture of microbes and yeast, it's extra important to avoid contamination.

Step 1: Make the tea

1. Make a full stockpot of tea, and leave it to brew for 15 to 20 minutes with the tea bags in it. Alternatively, add your tea to a saucepan of water and simmer it gently for 5 minutes.

2. Add the sugar and stir until it dissolves. Then add cool water to cool the tea. (You can add up to the same amount of water that might have evaporated during boiling.)

Note: Hot tea can kill the microbes in the scoby. The tea should be no warmer than body temperature when you add your starter.

Step 2: Make the brew

1. Pour the *cooled* tea into a bowl. Add the cider vinegar and the kombucha scoby. (You can order one online, buy it at a local health food store, or get one from a friend who makes kombucha.)

2. Put a tea towel over the bowl and secure it with a rubber band or a piece of elastic. This keeps contamination and insects out of your culture.

3. Put the bowl in a warm, dark place and leave it to ferment.

Step 3: Checking the brew

1. The fermentation will take 5 to 14 days, depending on the temperature. In warm climates 14 days is ample; in cold climates you may need 3 to 4 weeks. If you check your brew after 2 or 3 days, you'll notice a film forming on the surface. That's actually the first thin membrane of your new kombucha scoby—bacteria bred in your own kombucha.

2. Start tasting the brew after 4 or 5 days. It should have a tangy or sour taste. The longer you leave the scoby in it, the more sugar will be eaten by the microbes. So if it's still sweet, you know it's not quite ready.

Step 4: Bottling

1. When the kombucha is ready—a second scoby may be fully formed at the top of the liquid—gently lift the mother culture and its offspring out and put them onto a clean plate. Make sure your hands are clean to avoid contamination.

2. Strain the kombucha into the glass jug or bottles, leaving behind about 1 cup in the bowl as a starter for the next batch.

3. Now fill clean jar or bottles with the kombucha and seal with an airtight lid. Store the jar or bottles in the fridge.

4. Use one of the scobys for your next batch. You can make double the amount or give the scoby to a friend. It can be stored at room temperature in a small amount of tea (don't let it dry out). You'll notice it has thickened up and is now a creamy color, rather than transparent.

SAUERKRAUT

Sauerkraut is a classic fermented vegetable that makes a great addition to many meals and will also reduce your sugar cravings. If you crave sugar, eat a spoonful of sauerkraut and you'll find that it dissipates quite quickly.

Ingredients

1 head green or red cabbage

1 tablespoon sea salt

If you need extra brine:

1 additional tablespoon sea salt

4 cups unchlorinated water

Directions

1. Wash the cabbage and remove any spoiled outer leaves.

2. Remove the core and slice the cabbage into thin, uniform strips.

3. Place the strips in a large bowl, and sprinkle the sea salt over the top.

4. Allow it to sit for 15 minutes or so, and then start mashing it with your hands or with a mallet. The goal is to release the juices inside the leaves. Mash/knead for roughly 5 to 10 minutes. You'll now have salty cabbage juice sitting in the bottom of your bowl.

5. Place a couple of handfuls of cabbage into the jar, then thoroughly pack them down with a wooden spoon, eliminating as many air bubbles as possible. Repeat and pack tightly until the jar is nearly full, leaving about 2 inches at the top.

Note: There should be enough cabbage liquid to cover the contents. If there isn't, make a 2 percent brine solution to fill the rest of the jar. (If you don't completely submerge the cabbage in liquid, it may spoil.)

How to make a 2 percent brine:

1. Dissolve 1 tablespoon sea salt in 4 cups unchlorinated water. (Note: finer salt tends to dissolve faster.) If you don't use all of the brine for this recipe, it will keep indefinitely in the fridge.

2. Cover the exposed cabbage with cabbage juice or brine, covering all protruding leaves and leaving 1 inch of head space at the top.

3. Put the lid on the jar and tighten it very gently (use your fingers, not your wrist). Set aside at room temperature, out of direct sunlight, for at least 1 week.

Pro tip: You'll probably want to place a small dish or tray under the jar, as they have a tendency to leak a bit and spill over. In fact, it helps to remove the lid after a day or so to release any pent-up gases.

Group 3—Dairy

As we've learned, dairy has long been a staple in the diets of cultures all over the world. People have consumed milk, cheese, and butter from cows, goats, sheep, camels, and other animals for thousands of years.

But the dairy that's available to us today is very different from the dairy our ancestors drank and cooked with.

Lactose intolerance

People who lack the enzyme lactase—which lets us digest lactose, the sugar naturally found in milk—are said to be lactose intolerant. Two hours after consuming lactose, these people may experience symptoms including abdominal pain, bloating or cramps, diarrhea, gas, or nausea.[1]

If you are one of these people, you will need to avoid dairy containing lactose.

Casein intolerance

Along with whey, caseins are one of the main proteins naturally found in milk. Different kinds of dairy products have different levels of casein, and some people have trouble digesting it.

Symptoms of casein intolerance include:

- Diarrhea, constipation, gas, and bloating
- Headaches and migraines
- Dermatitis, skin allergies, and eczema
- Blocked sinuses and asthma

Casein intolerance may be due the homogenization and pasteurization of dairy products. This processing may strip these products of the enzymes that our gut bacteria need to digest casein. When casein-intolerant people balance their microbiome and stick to organic, unprocessed dairy products, they may find that casein is no longer a problem.

If you experience any of the above symptoms after eating dairy, you should try a period without dairy in your diet entirely. Reach for the other food groups in this tier—meats, fish, and fermented foods—to make sure you get enough A, D, and K2 in your diet. If your symptoms subside, then you may have a casein protein intolerance.

If you want to reintroduce dairy back into your life, it's important to understand the different forms of dairy and their different levels of lactose and casein.

Milk
Milk naturally contains both lactose and casein proteins; 250 milliliters of milk contain roughly 15 grams of lactose.

Yogurt and kefir
Both yogurt and kefir are made by putting bacterial colonies *back* into milk. The microbes digest some of the lactose in the milk and make these dairy products more digestible.

Yogurt has roughly 9.6 grams of lactose per 200 milliliters and is high in casein.

Kefir is 4 percent lactose but can have less lactose depending on the fermentation process.

Cheese
Cheeses generally have a very low level of lactose (0.4 percent), but cheese curd is formed by the coagulation of casein protein, so people with casein issues can have trouble with certain cheeses.

Milk fats
If you have lactose and casein problems, it's best to consume milk fats rather than milk because they contain the least lactose and casein.

Ghee—Ghee is made by simmering butter to clarify it, separating the proteins and sugar from the pure butterfat, which gives it the lowest levels of casein.

Butter—Butter has a little more lactose and casein than ghee.

Sour cream—Since it's fermented, sour cream has less lactose than cream.

Cream—Cream has the most lactose and casein of all the milk fats.

If you have removed dairy from your diet and you want to add it back in, you should always reintroduce ghee as a first step. You can then reintroduce butter, cream, cheese, yogurt, and milk, in that order.

HOMEMADE GHEE

Ghee is made by clarifying butter to remove the milk solids and leave the pure dairy fat.

Equipment
Saucepan

Fine wire mesh strainer

Cheesecloth

Spoon

16-ounce or larger measuring cup

Glass jar

Ingredients
16 ounces (1 pound) butter from grass-fed cows, cubed

Directions
1. Melt the butter in a saucepan over medium heat.
2. Bring the butter to a simmer.

3. Cook for about 10 to 15 minutes. During this time, watch it closely: First the surface will foam, then bubble, then almost stop bubbling, and then foam again. At this point, the butter should be a bright gold, with reddish solids on the bottom of the pan. This means the ghee is done.

4. Cool and then slowly pour the ghee through the wire mesh strainer lined with several layers of cheesecloth. The small bits of milk protein are usually discarded (though a friend told me that her grandmother used to mix those with flour, or almond flour, and a small bit of honey to make a flavorful fudgelike treat).

5. Ghee will last up to a month at room temperature, but it's better to store it in the fridge.

TIER 3

FATS AND OILS; NUTS, SEEDS, AND SPICES

Group 1—Fats and oils

Every meal—however it's prepared—should have fat. But this means natural fats, not processed or refined fats. As a guide, begin with 1 to 2 tablespoons of your choice of fat to use as a cooking base.

While known as saturated fats, the following fats actually contain higher percentages of monounsaturated fats (except for tallow, which has a higher percentage of saturated fats). Animal fats are excellent for all types of cooking. They include:

Animal fats (solid at room temperature)

- Chicken fat
- Lard (pig fat)
- Duck and goose fat
- Tallow (beef fat)

Oils (liquid at room temperature)

- Olive oil: Use extra-virgin and cold-pressed (mainly served cold).
- Sesame oil: High in omega-6s, so limit to 1 to 2 teaspoons per day.
- Flaxseed oil: Keep refrigerated, never heat, and limit to 1 to 2 teaspoons per day.
- Coconut oil: Has a high saturated fat content and is great for cooking; eat approximately 3 to 4 tablespoons per day.
- Palm oil: Use red, unprocessed palm oil.
- Avocado oil: Good for cooking (because it has heat-resistant properties) and for adding to salads.

Dairy fats

- Butter: Excellent addition for taste.
- Ghee: Great for cooking.

NON-FLOUR GRAVY

The beauty of incorporating fat into your diet is that it means there's no waste when you cook. For instance, a very tasty way to consume natural fats is to take fatty drippings and lumpy parts from cooking and turn them into gravy.

Equipment

Blender

Ingredients

3 cups fresh fatty drippings

¼ to ½ cup full cream or unsweetened coconut milk

2 tablespoons arrowroot powder or tapioca flour

Sea salt or rock salt to taste

Ground black pepper

1 pinch dried sage or any herb of your choice

Directions

1. Pour hot drippings into a saucepan. Add the cream, arrowroot powder, salt, pepper, and sage.

2. Pour the mixture into a blender and blend until smooth.

3. Pour it back into the saucepan and heat on low while stirring until the gravy thickens. Don't boil. (If it comes to a full rolling boil, the fat could separate out.) Season to taste.

4. If the gravy is too thin, add a bit of arrowroot powder to the warm mixture on the stove very slowly, using a fine mesh strainer and stirring briskly with a whisk to avoid lumps. If it's too thick, stir in a bit more drippings or cream. Serve immediately.

Group 2—Nuts, seeds, and spices

Add a handful or sprinkle of nuts, seeds, and spices to your meals, or eat nuts and seeds as snacks.

Nuts

- Almonds
- Walnuts
- Pecans
- Pine nuts
- Brazil nuts
- Cashews

Seeds

Seeds are great sources of zinc, magnesium, fats, and many other phytochemicals.

- Pumpkin
- Sunflower
- Sesame
- Chia
- Flax

Spices

Spices are rich in phytonutrients. Every meal is an opportunity to add spices, either while you cook or on the plate.

- Sea salt or pink rock salt (avoid refined table salt)
- Pepper
- Cardamom
- Turmeric
- Cayenne
- Cinnamon
- Cloves
- Ginger
- Nutmeg

TIER 4

FRUITS AND GRAINS

Fruits

Our body is generally designed to consume fructose in 2 or 3 small pieces of fruit per day. (The problem is that most people take in extra sugar from a lot of other sources.) Avoid fruit juices altogether—they're a concentrated hit of sugar. And limit how much fruit you put in your smoothies.

Low-fructose fruits you can eat more often

- Kiwifruit
- Blueberries and raspberries
- Grapefruit
- Lemons/limes
- Honeydew melon
- Pear
- Coconut
- Avocado

Higher-fructose fruits to eat sparingly

- Grapes
- Cherries
- Pineapple
- Watermelon
- Raisins
- Prunes
- Dates
- All other dried fruit

Grains

Limit to 2 or 3 servings per week, and stick to whole-grain varieties that have been fermented, sprouted, or soaked, such as:

- Barley
- Brown/black rice
- Buckwheat
- Oatmeal
- Millet
- Sourdough
- Sprouted bread
- Dark rye bread

REMEMBER TO ENJOY YOUR FOOD!

If you follow the guidelines and stick to the foods above, you'll keep your mouth, teeth, and entire body healthy. It won't happen overnight, but if you keep at it, it will happen.

And remember, eating healthy is about eating the *right* food, much more than the right *amount* of food. It's important to try to stick to the servings recommended above, but your first priority should be to eat a rich variety of foods, properly sourced and prepared, from all of the groups above.

After you cook and eat these foods more and get to know where they come from, this will all become second nature to you. And if you stick to the food groups, your portions will become second nature as well.

It will take some time, to be sure. But you'll notice a difference in how you feel sooner rather than later. And before you know it, eating according to the principles of the Dental Diet will lead to the most painless visits to the dentist you've ever had.

CHAPTER 11

THE 40-DAY DENTAL DIET MEAL PLAN

As I began to adopt the Dental Diet, it seemed like everything I had previously eaten was unhealthy. At times it was overwhelming. When I felt that way, I reminded myself that there are usually no shortcuts when you want to make a significant change to your life. The Dental Diet is no different.

At the same time, I felt like I was going through a rebirth. I discovered a world of new, fresher foods, and as my taste buds awoke, I rediscovered flavors in foods I had not eaten for a large portion of my life. I experimented with new ways of cooking and had new and healthier cravings. Different foods started to taste good together—it was thrilling. It wasn't always easy, but it was definitely always rewarding.

To develop a proper diet, one that other people could adopt, I had to collect and create a lot of dishes and recipes. They had to check all the boxes in the principles for good dental nutrition, and they had to be tasty. I wanted to take advantage of traditional cooking techniques, but the recipes had to be practical and time-efficient, too. Otherwise, the diet would never stick. It took a lot of experimenting, but after some time I learned which dishes need a bit more care and time and which can be prepared quickly and easily.

After it was "ready," I recommended the diet to my family and friends. They gave me positive feedback, and eventually, alongside dietary analysis, I brought it into my dental practice. Patients who took up the plan saw improvements to their dental health and overall health very quickly. The biggest challenges they experienced were removing sugar from their diet and learning cooking techniques that were centuries old but new to them.

I've laid out the following 40-day meal plan to take all of the guesswork out for you. It's designed to make sure that your body gets just the right amount of the nutrients, microbes, and other dietary factors we've talked about. It will also make your food buying and preparation a lot simpler. You can hit the ground running. Soon you'll acquire healthy eating habits that should last a lifetime.

I understand that many people won't be able to do *everything* I outline in this plan. That's absolutely fine. Do what you can, knowing the more you follow the principles of the diet, the healthier your mouth and body will be.

PREVIEW

Week 1

Removing processed food

In the first week, you'll start with the first of the three major steps of the program. You'll *eliminate* packaged, processed, and refined foods from your diet (and begin to understand how you can live without them).

Weeks 2 and 3

Going sugar-free and staying strong

In week one, you removed all the sugar that comes with processed foods. In weeks two and three, you'll cut all the sugar that comes from fruits. This will give your body a chance to completely balance the microbial communities in your mouth and gut and relieve your liver of the metabolic burden of fructose.

It's not going to be easy, but freeing yourself from the grip of sugar will be worth it. By the end of these two weeks, you'll notice that your palate will have significantly changed, and any small amount of sugar will taste extremely—and perhaps unnecessarily—sweet!

Week 4

Reintroducing fruit and bringing in fasting

After you've established a sturdy microbiome and a metabolism that no longer depends on sugar, you can reintroduce whole fruit into your diet. Without the constant need for the instant gratification of simple carbs, you'll be able to fast for two to three meals per week—I recommend breakfast—to allow your microbiome and metabolism to heal even more.

Weeks 5 and 6

Reintroducing restaurant foods and your new normal

Nothing in life should be too rigid, and that includes our diet. In the final period of the program, you can begin to reintroduce restaurant food. (Though you don't *have* to!) Besides, if the Dental Diet didn't allow a little splurging now and then, you'd be much less likely to follow it, and I certainly don't want anyone to give up their social life, including (and especially) myself! By now, you'll also have settled into a new way of seeing food, and the new cooking methods you've learned will be second nature.

THE PROGRAM

Dietary Supplements

As you embark upon the program, it's important to make sure your body has enough of the three main fat-soluble vitamins—A, D, and K2—as well as their support nutrients. They'll aid your dental healing and, of course, your overall health. The following supplemental foods will make sure you get them.

Vitamin A

Extra-virgin cod-liver oil: Take daily, as directed on the package. (**Warning:** You should always read labels and stick to recommended dosages of cod-liver oil to prevent an overdose of vitamin A.)

Vitamin D

Sunlight: Our bodies synthesize vitamin D from sunlight, so the best supplement for vitamin D is spending 30 minutes a day in sunlight whenever possible. Cod-liver oil is the best natural alternate source. Some people will additionally need a vitamin D supplement; be sure to talk to your doctor and get your blood levels checked to address your personal needs.

Vitamin K2

Emu oil or high-vitamin butter oil: To make sure you're getting enough of the crucial vitamin K2, you can take high-vitamin butter oil or emu oil in capsules (as directed), or 1 teaspoon per day, *after* the largest meal of the day. For supplementation you can take 150 to 200 milligrams of MK7 vitamin K2. (**Warning:** If you take warfarin, you should talk with your doctor before supplementing or changing your intake of vitamin K1 or K2.)

Gelatin

If you don't have time to cook your own bone broth, you can buy collagen powder. Make sure it's sourced from grass-raised animals. Mix it with soup or hot water.

Apple cider vinegar
This is one of the easiest fermented foods to obtain. You can buy it from almost any grocery store. Add it cold to salads or add a tablespoon to a glass of water. (Take one "dose" per day for better digestion.)

Food Prep

Homemade chicken or beef broth
You'll add this broth to meals when you can. One cup a day is great. (Recipes appear in Chapter 10.)

Tip: If you can't cook beef broth, add collagen powder to soups or hot water.

Homemade fermented food prep of your choice
Shoot for 2 to 3 small servings per day of sauerkraut, kefir, or kombucha. (See recipes in Chapter 10.)

Dairy Intolerance
If you experience symptoms of dairy intolerance, replace dairy products with almond milk, coconut milk, coconut yogurt, or coconut kefir when possible.

Snack Ideas
The 40-day meal plan will leave you feeling full, satisfied, and without cravings or energy crashes. Remember you're not calorie counting, so if you do feel a hunger pang between meals, your main mission is to avoid refined, sugary foods that promote blood sugar spikes and tooth decay. The following ideas are great ways to fill a void and will keep you feeling content. Limit snacks that contain natural sugars to one per day. Snacks that are sugar-free can be enjoyed to your heart's content!

Sugar-free options
- Boiled eggs
- Salted avocado
- Coconut chips
- Nuts
- Hummus with carrots/celery
- Cheese and pâté
- Raw carrots/celery

Sugar included
- Berries
- Whole fruit

WEEK 1: REMOVING PROCESSED FOOD

Our bodies are not designed to use the simple carbs and artificial compounds that tend to make up most processed foods. So eliminating them from your diet will automatically help your body function better.

How you'll feel
In this week, you'll generally feel more energized. By removing processed foods, you'll remove the burden that your body has to carry to break them down. You'll also feel an immediate difference from getting the right amount of fat-soluble vitamins. Some people feel guilty for eating tasty, full-fat foods, but these are foods your body needs (contrary to what you might have assumed). Enjoy them!

In this stage we'll also replace processed sugars with natural ones, which will help lessen sugar cravings and withdrawal during the next phase of the program.

Before you eat, you breathe

The Dental Diet is focused on making sure that your body receives the nutrients it needs the most. We can't forget that oxygen is at the top of that list as your body's most essential nutrient. Each week you'll do daily breathing, tongue, or voice exercises to help strengthen your mouth, airways, and breathing habits, thereby improving the oxygenation of your body. With these simple, two- to three-minute exercises, you'll give yourself better breathing habits that will last your whole life.

Before you eat: Breathing Exercise

Note: Each *Before you eat* exercise will benefit you the most if you do it before meals, because it will help prepare your digestive system to make the most of the nutrients you take in. But really, the exercises are great at any time of the day or night.

Diaphragmatic Breathing Exercises (once before each meal)

Slower, deeper breathing allows your body to extract more oxygen from the air. It also activates your parasympathetic nervous system, which helps your digestive system to function at its peak.

This exercise is designed to help you use your diaphragmatic muscles when you breathe in. Your belly should expand instead of your chest. (When you breathe into your belly by contracting your diaphragm, it maximizes the space for your lungs to expand to and take in air.)

1. Sit with a straight back and your mouth closed. Put one hand over your belly and relax your shoulders, jaw, and neck.

2. Breathe in for three seconds, letting your belly expand. When you inhale, you should feel your hand being pushed forward by the expansion of your belly.

> 3. Then breathe out for four seconds, releasing the air through your nose. Your hand should move back toward you, as you pull your belly back toward your spine. Repeat the cycle 20 times (three seconds in, four seconds out).
>
> If you have trouble, keep practicing. It takes time to learn to use these muscle groups to breathe this way.

FOOD PROGRAM

Day 1

Breakfast: Banana and 1 tablespoon of coconut oil with soaked black chia seeds, almonds, and one scoop of sheep's milk yogurt topped with cinnamon. Serve with a side of kefir.

Lunch: Scrambled eggs with red peppers, turmeric, and feta cheese. Serve with a side of sauerkraut.

Dinner:

RED BUTTER ROAST BEEF

Serves 4

Ingredients

4 tablespoons butter, melted	1 bunch fresh thyme, chopped
2 medium onions, chopped	3 tablespoons sea salt
1 whole broccoli, chopped	1 tablespoon cayenne pepper
1 clove garlic, chopped	1 tablespoon paprika
2 carrots, chopped	3.3 pounds topside of beef

Directions

1. Preheat oven to 475°F.

2. Place onions, broccoli, garlic, carrots, and thyme in the middle of a large roasting tray.

3. Combine butter with salt, cayenne, and paprika in a small bowl.

4. Drizzle beef with about three-quarters of the butter mixture and place on vegetables.

5. Turn oven down to 400° and place the roast inside. Every 20 minutes, baste the beef and vegetables with leftover butter to prevent drying. Cook for 60 minutes for medium doneness. For medium rare, reduce cooking time by 10 to 15 minutes. For well done, cook 10 to 15 minutes more.

6. Place any leftovers in the fridge for snacks or a savory breakfast.

Dessert: 1 piece whole fruit.

Day 2

Breakfast: Yogurt topped with berries and walnuts. Serve with coffee or tea.

Lunch: Roasted pumpkin, fennel, and quinoa salad with thyme, oregano, olive oil, and butter. Serve with a side of kefir.

Dinner:

SALMON HEAD SOUP

Serves 2

Ingredients

2 carrots, chopped

2 stalks celery, chopped

1 onion

1 bunch dill

2 bay leaves

2 whole salmon heads

Directions

1. Add all ingredients to a large pot and just barely cover with filtered water. Add a sprinkle of sea salt and white vinegar for flavor.

2. Cook for 20 minutes and then remove the fish heads.

3. Remove cooked flesh from the fish heads and serve separately, or place back in the soup.

4. Leftover soup can be kept in the fridge for 2 to 3 days.

Dessert: Warmed coconut oil with crushed nuts, berries, cinnamon, and a sprinkle of salt.

Day 3

Breakfast: Chive, kale, and parmesan scrambled eggs cooked in butter and served with a side of sauerkraut.

Lunch: Chicken or duck pâté and a hard cheese platter. Serve with a tossed mixed green salad dressed with olive oil.

Dinner:

ITALIAN-STYLE CHICKEN DRUMSTICKS

Serves 3 to 4

Ingredients

Olive oil

6 to 8 chicken thighs and/or drumsticks

2 to 3 cloves garlic, chopped

Paprika

Sea salt

Pepper

4 tomatoes, chopped

1 green pepper, chopped

½ cup green olives

3 to 4 tablespoons fresh oregano

1 cup dried chickpea pasta

Directions

1. Preheat oven to 375°F.

2. Coat a baking pan with olive oil. Add chicken and chopped garlic and sprinkle with paprika, sea salt, and pepper.

3. Cook chicken for 20 minutes until brown.

4. Remove chicken from oven, turn, and add tomatoes, green pepper, olives, oregano, and additional salt and pepper.

5. Bake for another half hour, until cooked through.

6. Remove from the oven to turn legs and mix sauce.

7. Bring a pot of salted water to a boil. Add chickpea pasta and cook for 20 minutes.

8. Serve chicken dish over the pasta. Pair with a glass of organic red wine and the leftover fish soup from last night.

Dessert: A few squares of dark (85 to 90 percent) chocolate with almonds.

Day 4

Breakfast: Shaved coconut with yogurt, walnuts, and diced apple, topped with cinnamon. Optional coffee or tea.

Lunch: Tuna, hard-boiled egg, and avocado salad with baby spinach and pickled onions drizzled with olive oil.

Dinner:

BEEF LIVER STEAK

Serves 2

Ingredients

1 sweet potato

2 tablespoons ghee, butter, coconut oil, melted lard, or tallow

3 teaspoons salt

1 to 2 fillets of beef liver

1 bunch fresh oregano

1 tablespoon fresh chopped ginger

1 red chili pepper, chopped

1 lime

Directions

1. Preheat oven to 400°F.

2. Cut sweet potato into strips. Place in roasting pan, adding 1 tablespoon of ghee and salt.

3. Place in oven for 30 minutes or until soft.

4. Put remaining ghee in a frying pan on medium heat.

5. Add beef liver, oregano, ginger, chili, and lime and cook until liver is tender. Be careful not to cook for too long or liver will become tough.

6. Serve liver steak and sweet potato fries with juices from the roasting pan and with kombucha.

Day 5

Breakfast: Fried eggs with bacon, cooked in lard or coconut oil, with sliced avocado and a side of kefir.

Lunch: Watercress salad, cucumber pasta with olive oil, and sauerkraut.

Dinner:

WHOLE CHICKEN BROTH

Serves 4

Ingredients

1 whole chicken

2 carrots, chopped

1 onion

2 stalks celery, chopped

2 tablespoons vinegar

1 teaspoon whole peppercorns

1 bunch fresh thyme

2 to 3 teaspoons sea salt

Directions

1. Follow the directions for Chicken Broth in Chapter 10 (page 209).

2. Boil, then reduce heat and simmer for 2 to 6 hours.

3. Drain, cool, and serve. Eat leftover chicken with broth and store any leftover broth in fridge or freezer.

4. Serve with ginger tea.

Dessert: Yogurt topped with berries.

Day 6

Breakfast: Kefir with flaxseed (soaked for 2 minutes in 1 tablespoon of warmed coconut oil), banana, almonds, and cinnamon.

Lunch: Beef mince stir-fry with onions, garlic, mushrooms, and broccolini. Serve with a cup of last night's broth.

Dinner: Grilled cold-water fish (e.g., tuna, herring, or salmon) of your choice, served with a side of sauerkraut, steamed asparagus, and optional glass of red wine.

Dessert: Sliced apples fried in coconut oil, topped with cinnamon.

Day 7

Breakfast: Bacon and eggs with roasted potatoes, served with cream on top and green tea.

Lunch: Raw chopped vegetable salad of cabbage, carrots, and celery, dressed with olive oil and balsamic vinegar. Kefir on the side.

Dinner:

CHEESY MEXICAN BEEF STIR-FRY

Serves 4

Ingredients

1 tablespoon lard, tallow, or ghee

2 cloves garlic, minced

1 teaspoon of cumin

1 teaspoon of oregano

1 pound top steak, cut into thin strips

1 onion, chopped

1 red bell pepper, cut into thin strips

1 or 2 jalapeño peppers, seeded and sliced thin

10 ounces brie cheese, chopped and removed from rind

2 avocados

1 lime

3 cups shredded iceberg lettuce

Directions

1. Heat lard in a pan over medium heat. Add garlic, cumin, oregano, and beef strips and cook until browned.

2. Add onion, bell pepper, and jalapeño to pan.

3. When onion is browned, add brie to the pan and heat to melt.

4. Cut and mash avocados, squeeze lime and serve with lettuce on side of spiced steak and cheese mixture.

Dessert: Small glass of organic wine or unpasteurized beer.

WEEK 2: GOING SUGAR-FREE

In week 1, we cut your sugar intake dramatically. But at the same time, you were eating natural forms of sugar that came mainly from fruits. The next two weeks are designed to take you to the next level and cut out sugar altogether.

How you'll feel
This is the most challenging part of the program. In most cases, people will experience a roller coaster of cravings or other general discomfort. For some, this will last three or four days, but for others it can last the entire two weeks. It may be tough, but it's more than worth it. After these two weeks, your body will recognize the foods that it *needs* instead of the sugary foods it's been conditioned to crave.

Rule: Eat no refined sugar or natural sources of sugar (such as fruits). Many diets recommend removing only refined sugar from the diet. But for these next two weeks, we're excluding all artificial sweeteners *and* natural sweeteners from our diet.

Make sure to remove all foods or sugar additives during weeks 2 and 3, including:

- Fruit
- Honey
- Agave nectar
- Brown sugar
- Coconut sugar
- Corn sweetener
- Molasses
- Maple syrup
- Stevia

How to beat sugar cravings

If a sugar craving sets in, try one of the following antidotes to keep yourself from reaching for a sugary treat.

- 1 tablespoon coconut oil: The medium-chain triglycerides in coconut oil will be absorbed quickly into your bloodstream, and this often stems sugar cravings.
- 1 tablespoon of melted butter: Good, old-fashioned butter! It helps you feel satisfied with a vitamin-rich dose of fat.
- 1 tablespoon sauerkraut: Even though it's not very sweet, sauerkraut helps reverse the body's craving for sugar.
- 1 handful spiced nuts, especially Brazil nuts, which are high in selenium, an element that reduces cravings for sweets.
- 1 handful coconut chips.
- A hot (or cold) shower. Resetting your body temperature can often disrupt the cycle of craving.
- Exercise! Go for a walk, run, or do 10 push-ups, jumping jacks, or star jumps.
- Green tea or peppermint tea.
- Diaphragmatic breathing exercise (from week 1).

Food prep for the week

Most of the times we make bad food choices, it's because we lack better options. Getting food ready in advance for the entire week is a great way to avoid this problem. It will mean that something healthy is always on hand.

Here are some great recipes to replace anything sugary that you may be reaching for.

NUT BREAD

Equipment

1 8" x 4" bread tin

Ingredients

4 to 5 cups mixed walnuts, almonds, and pecans

2 cups mixed seeds—pumpkin, sunflower, chia, and flaxseed

5 eggs

¼ cup olive oil

1 teaspoon sea salt

Directions

1. Preheat oven to 320°F.

2. Chop nuts and seeds, or place in a blender and pulse lightly. Then put them in a mixing bowl.

3. Mix eggs, oil, and salt in a separate bowl. Once mixed, combine with nuts and seeds.

4. Grease a bread tin with olive oil, then spread the batter evenly in the tin.

5. Bake for 60 minutes or until the bread is firm. Let it cool, then cut into slices.

PICKLED GINGER

Equipment

Wide-mouth glass jar

Ingredients

3- to 4-inch fresh ginger root, peeled and thinly sliced

2 tablespoons sea salt

Directions

1. Place ginger in a bowl and pound with a rounded utensil to release juice. Transfer to a jar with a lid.

2. Add salt and enough water to cover ginger (leaving 1 inch at the top of the jar).

3. Screw lid on and keep for 3 to 4 days at room temperature to let it ferment before transferring to refrigerator for storage.

Before you eat: Tongue Exercise (once before each meal)

This exercise will help hold your tongue at the top of your mouth while you rest, which will help the muscles stay active at night. It will also help your breathing and digestion.

Hold your tongue just behind your back teeth, just behind the two grooves on your palate. Close your lips, breathe through your nose, and push upward with your tongue, including the back of the tongue. Hold for three minutes.

Day 8

Breakfast: Spinach, potato, and fresh oregano scrambled eggs, cooked in coconut oil or ghee and served with nut bread and kefir.

Lunch: Pickled ginger and lime tuna salad with arugula, topped with fresh mint and olive oil. Serve with a side of kombucha.

Dinner:

MOROCCAN LAMB

Serves 4

Ingredients

Lard or tallow

Lamb shoulder

1 onion, chopped

2 red or green peppers, chopped

1 teaspoon turmeric

1 teaspoon ginger

1 teaspoon cumin

1 teaspoon paprika

1 teaspoon chili powder

2 tomatoes, chopped

1 tablespoon tomato paste

1 cup chickpeas

1 cup beef stock

Sea salt to taste

Pepper to taste

Directions

1. Heat fat in a saucepan over medium heat.

2. Cook lamb shoulder in pan until browned. Remove and set aside.

3. Add onion and peppers to the same pan and cook until soft. Add turmeric, ginger, cumin, paprika, and chili powder, and stir until fragrant.

4. Add tomatoes, tomato paste, and chickpeas to pan. Cook for 1 minute before returning lamb to pan. Add beef stock, cook, and stir on low heat for 10 to 15 minutes. Season with salt and pepper to taste, and serve in bowls.

Dessert: Nuts coated in cinnamon and vanilla extract (make sure there is no *added* sugar) in warm coconut oil.

Day 9

Breakfast: Avocado, feta, and cilantro smash on nut bread with olive oil. Serve with kefir.

Lunch: Liver pâté with hard cheese platter.

Dinner: Beef, pork, or lamb sausages pan-fried in lard, served with beef or chicken stock gravy, sweet potato, and carrot chips in butter. Add a glass of kombucha on the side.

Day 10

Breakfast:

HOMEMADE GRANOLA

Serves 6

Ingredients

½ cup chopped almonds

½ cup sunflower seeds

½ cup pumpkin seeds

½ cup shredded coconut

1 teaspoon ground cinnamon

1 teaspoon sea salt

1 teaspoon vanilla extract

2 tablespoons coconut oil

Directions

1. Preheat oven to 300°F.

2. Mix all ingredients in a bowl with clean hands and place on a baking tray.

3. Bake for 10 to 15 minutes, until browned. Serve with full-fat yogurt.

4. Store leftovers in an airtight container.

Lunch: Chopped raw salad bowl with celery, carrots, and soft-boiled eggs, topped with olive oil and salt. Serve with a side of kombucha.

Dinner:

ZESTY PEPPER CHICKEN WINGS WITH SWEET POTATO CHIPS AND GUACAMOLE

Serves 2 to 3

Ingredients

2 tablespoons lemon zest (from 3 to 4 lemons)

1 teaspoon salt, or to taste

1 tablespoon freshly cracked black pepper

¼ cup ghee, melted

2 pounds chicken wings

1 sweet potato, diced

2 avocados, pitted, peeled, and minced

1 tablespoon lemon juice

Directions

1. Preheat oven to 375°F.

2. Combine lemon zest, salt, pepper, and half of the ghee in a bowl. Season chicken wings with half of the mixture and transfer to a roasting pan.

3. Add diced sweet potato and top all with the last half of ghee and salt.

4. Add avocado and lemon juice. Stir until mixed.

5. Bake chicken for 30 minutes, until cooked through.

6. Serve warm with guacamole on the side.

Sugar-free snack:

SPICED NUTS

Equipment

Baking tray

Ingredients

2 cups nuts (choose from a mix of almonds, cashews, walnuts, pecans, and pumpkin seeds)

3 tablespoons coconut oil

1 teaspoon of mixed spices of your choice

1 teaspoon cinnamon

Directions

1. Preheat oven to 300°F.

2. Place nuts on tray and top with coconut oil and spices.

3. Bake for 10 to 15 minutes until brown.

4. Store in an airtight jar.

Day 11
Breakfast:

GREEN FRITTATA

Serves 2

Ingredients

3 green onions	1 handful pepitas
2 zucchini	2 tablespoons of coconut oil or lard
1 bunch baby spinach	6 eggs
1 bunch basil, chopped	½ cup cream
1 bunch parsley, chopped	2 tablespoons extra-virgin olive oil
2 cloves garlic, chopped	

Directions

1. Chop green onions, zucchini, and spinach into roughly even, small pieces.

2. Cook basil, parsley, green onions, zucchini, spinach, garlic, and pepitas in coconut oil or lard in medium-size sauté pan for 5 minutes, until lightly softened.

3. Whisk in eggs. Cook for 2 to 3 minutes and turn over until both sides are brown. Add cream and olive oil, and pour over cooked vegetables. Spice to taste.

Lunch: Pan-fried salmon and kale topped with butter, with a side of sauerkraut.

Dinner:

FENNEL AND LEEK HOT POT

Serves 3 to 4

Ingredients

1 tablespoon lard, coconut oil, or ghee

2 leeks, chopped

2 stalks celery, chopped

2 white onions, chopped

1 bulb fennel, chopped

3 cups beef or chicken broth

2 tablespoons salt

1 bunch cilantro, chopped

2 sprigs fresh thyme, chopped

Directions

1. Heat lard in a saucepan over high heat.

2. Cook leeks, celery, onions, and fennel in saucepan, tossing occasionally, until brown, about 8 to 10 minutes.

3. Pour broth into saucepan and add salt, cilantro, thyme, and other spices to taste.

4. Serve with butter and nut bread.

Day 12

Breakfast: Sautéed brussels sprouts and mushrooms served with sour cream and chives.

Lunch: Guacamole spread with fried egg, served on nut bread.

Dinner: Oven-baked white fish fillet with bok choy, served with kombucha.

Dessert:

AVOCADO MOUSSE

Ingredients

2 ripe avocados

½ cup cream

½ cup raw cacao powder

1 teaspoon vanilla extract

1 teaspoon cinnamon

Pinch of salt

Directions

1. Place ingredients in blender, process until smooth.

2. Serve cold in a bowl with full cream or as a spread on nut bread.

Day 13

Breakfast: Soft-boiled eggs with onions, diced tomato, sage, and cayenne pepper.

Lunch: Pan-fried chicken with chopped chili, served with cold potato and green bean salad.

Dinner:

ORGAN MEATBALLS WITH CUCUMBER PASTA

Serves 4

Ingredients

1 pound ground meat of your choice; include 2 slices liver meat, chopped

1 cup of vegetable pasta (page 203)

1 egg

1 bunch parsley

3 cloves garlic

1 bunch basil

1 diced tomato

1 bunch oregano

1 bunch mint

1 tablespoon sea salt

Pepper to taste

Directions

1. Preheat oven to 350°F.

2. Place all ingredients in a bowl and mix until consistent. Form into balls.

3. Place on baking tray lined with wax paper and bake for 20 to 25 minutes.

4. Place 2 or 3 meatballs on top of cucumber pasta and serve warm. (Save leftovers for a quick and easy breakfast or lunch later in the week.)

Day 14

Breakfast:

ISRAELI-STYLE EGGS

Serves 2

Ingredients

1 onion, chopped

1 bell pepper, chopped

1 cup tomato paste

1 bunch parsley

4 eggs

Directions

1. Sauté chopped onion, bell peppers, tomato paste, and parsley in pan for 5 to 7 minutes.

2. Crack eggs into pan, cover, and cook for 5 to 10 minutes on medium heat.

3. Sprinkle with fresh parsley and serve in hot pan.

Lunch: San Choy Bao—iceberg lettuce leaves topped with meatball leftovers, grated peppers, and carrot.

Dinner: Pan-fried trout with broccoli and beef or chicken broth.

WEEK 3: STAYING STRONG

You're halfway through your sugar-free period. Stay strong! You've also made it through the hardest part of *The Dental Diet* 40-day program. Congratulations! (Time to celebrate with a shot of cod-liver oil!)

How you'll feel
The first seven days that you completely remove sugar from your diet make for a harsh learning experience for your body. But by Week 2, you may already be free of sugar cravings. Or you might still be craving sugar, but by the end of this week, this should completely subside. Your body will feel much more stable, and you'll no longer have those violent hunger pangs or dips in energy.

Before you eat: Alternate Nostril Breathing exercise (once before each meal)

This exercise will make you more comfortable breathing through your nose.

1. Sit with your back straight and shoulders back.

2. Block your right nostril and take a deep breath through your left nostril for 3 seconds.

3. Unblock your right nostril and block the left nostril, breathing out through the right nostril for 4 seconds.

4. Breathe in for 3 seconds through the right nostril.

5. Unblock your right nostril and breathe in through the left nostril.

6. Continue to cycle nostril breathing for 20 breaths (or approximately 3 minutes).

No-sugar dessert:

NUT-FUDGE CHOCOLATE BROWNIES

Serves 4

Ingredients

1 cup mashed sweet potato

½ cup warmed nut butter or alternative nut spread

½ cup cocoa powder (if you prefer a richer, stronger taste, you can add more cocoa)

1 teaspoon vanilla extract (make sure there's no added sugar)

1 teaspoon cinnamon

2 tablespoons butter

Directions

1. Preheat oven to 350°F.

2. Coat bread tin or cooking pan with butter.

3. Place all ingredients in a high-speed blender or food processor. Process until just blended.

4. Transfer batter to pan and bake for 12 to 15 minutes. Allow the brownies to cool in the pan completely before slicing into bars.

5. Serve topped with full cream.

Day 15

Breakfast: Soft-boiled eggs served with chopped fresh ginger and green onions, with kefir on the side.

Lunch: Rainbow bean salad: mung beans, fresh basil, red pepper, tomato, onion, and carrot, chopped and topped with fresh rosemary, olive oil, and salt.

Dinner: Lamb chops pan-fried in lard with squash, baby tomatoes, and broth.

Day 16

Breakfast: Asparagus wrapped in bacon and fried in duck fat, served with sauerkraut.

Lunch: Oven-roasted sesame- and chia-coated avocados and a green leafy salad dressed in olive oil, served with kombucha.

Dinner:

CREAMED CHICKEN LIVER PÂTÉ

Serves 2

Ingredients

½ cup ghee or butter

1 onion, chopped

1 pound chicken livers

½ cup cream

3 cloves garlic, chopped

1 ground clove

5 ground coriander seeds

Sea salt

1 tablespoon brandy

1 cucumber, sliced

Directions

1. Melt ghee in pan over medium-high heat.

2. Add onion and cook, stirring, until soft.

3. Add livers and cook on high heat for 2 minutes until browned on the outside.

4. Place livers, juice from pan, cream, spices, salt, and brandy in a blender. Puree until smooth.

5. Place in bowl and refrigerate for 2 to 3 hours.

6. Top each cucumber slice with pâté, and serve on a platter.

Day 17

Breakfast: Eggs cooked in butter and herbs, served on zucchini pasta.

Lunch: Fried sardines with a salad of arugula, parmesan, and capers.

Dinner: Oven-roasted lamb shanks in broth with bok choy, carrots, and onions.

Dessert: Nut-Fudge Brownies.

Day 18

Breakfast: Fried mushrooms stuffed with crispy bacon chips in butter.

Lunch: Cured meat platter with artichokes and sundried tomatoes.

Dinner:

CAULIFLOWER GRILLED CHEESE SANDWICH

Ingredients

1 head cauliflower, cut into small florets, stem removed

2 large eggs

½ cup Parmesan cheese, shredded

Sea salt

1 tablespoon oregano (or other spices of your choice)

17 ounces Gouda cheese, sliced

Lard or butter

Directions

1. Preheat oven to 450°F.

2. Pulse cauliflower in blender to a consistency similar to rice.

3. Transfer to a large bowl and cook cauliflower in a microwave for 5 minutes on high, intermittently removing to stir and even out. Repeat once until cauliflower is slightly moist and clumping. Cool for a few minutes.

4. Add eggs, parmesan, and salt. Stir until the mixture has a pasty consistency.

5. Lay the mixture in flat squares on a large baking sheet with parchment paper. Bake for 15 minutes, until browned.

6. Grease a pan with lard. Place sliced cheese between two cauliflower layers (to make a sandwich) and cook in the pan for 5 to 10 minutes, until cheese is melted.

Day 19
Breakfast:

AVOCADO EGG BOATS

Serves 2

Ingredients
2 avocados, halved

4 eggs

Chives

Cayenne pepper

Directions
1. Preheat oven to 420°F.

2. Place avocados on a roasting pan. Crack eggs into the space where the pit was.

3. Roast for 15 to 20 minutes. Remove and season with chives and cayenne.

4. Serve with sauerkraut.

Lunch:

COLESLAW

Serves 2

Ingredients

2 cups green and purple cabbage, finely shredded

2 cups carrot, shredded

¼ cup white vinegar (or apple cider vinegar)

2 cloves garlic

½ teaspoon sea salt

½ teaspoon black pepper

½ teaspoon dry mustard

½ teaspoon celery seed

½ cup mayonnaise

Directions

1. Mix cabbage and carrot in a bowl.

2. In a mixing cup, combine all other ingredients and whisk.

3. Add mayo mixture to cabbage and carrot and combine well, seasoning to taste. Serve with smoked salmon.

Dinner: Lamb or beef burger topped with mayonnaise, pickles, and tomato and wrapped in lettuce "buns."

Day 20

Breakfast: Soft poached eggs with ricotta cheese and pepitas.

Lunch: Meat patties coated with sesame seeds; zucchini chips on the side.

Dinner:

CLAM–CAULIFLOWER CHOWDER

Serves 4

Ingredients

2 tablespoon butter

2 cloves garlic, minced

1 onion, chopped

2 carrots, grated

1 head cauliflower, chopped

4 slices bacon

½ cup full cream or 1 cup milk

1 cup chicken stock

10 to 12 ounces fresh or canned clams

1 bunch fresh parsley, chopped

1 bay leaf

½ teaspoon turmeric

1 teaspoon cumin

Sea salt and freshly ground pepper

Directions

1. Melt butter in a large saucepan over medium heat. Add garlic, onion, and carrots. Cook until tender.

2. Stir in cauliflower and bacon, and cook for about 5 minutes.

3. Add cream, chicken stock, clams, parsley, bay leaf, and spices. Stir together.

4. Bring to a boil, then reduce heat and simmer for 15 minutes, until vegetables are tender. Season to taste.

Day 21

Breakfast: Spinach, kale, sunflower seeds, and scrambled eggs with butter.

Lunch: Cold tuna steak with arugula, pumpkin, and ginger salad.

Dinner:

OVEN-BAKED CURRY CHICKEN LEGS WITH SWEET POTATOES AND BROCCOLI

Serves 4

Ingredients

1 ½ teaspoons turmeric

1 tablespoon olive oil

6 to 8 chicken legs

½ sweet potato, chopped

1 head broccoli, chopped

1 teaspoon sea salt

1 teaspoon pepper

2 tablespoons butter, coconut oil, or animal fat, melted

Directions

1. Preheat oven to 400°F.

2. Combine turmeric and olive oil in a bowl. Coat chicken legs with this mixture and place them in a pan.

3. Add sweet potato and broccoli to pan, and top with salt, pepper, and butter.

4. Bake for 35 to 40 minutes or until brown.

5. Season to taste and serve in juice from pan.

WEEK 4: REINTRODUCING FRUIT AND BRINGING IN FASTING

You've made it three weeks without any added sugar! By this stage, your sugar cravings should largely be a thing of the past, and your energy levels should have stabilized. Now we will reintroduce whole fruit and introduce 12- to 14-hour fasts, where we simply skip breakfast two or three times a week to allow your body a rest from digestion.

How you'll feel
Your hunger cycles and energy should feel much more level and balanced. You should be sleeping better, too. When you do get

sweet cravings, you'll know what your "go-to" is to stay away from a sugary snack.

Before you eat: Tongue Strengthening Exercises (once before each meal)

These exercises will make the muscles along the side of your tongue and down your throat feel tired. That's good; it means you're training your muscles to chew and breathe properly.

1. Tap your tongue behind your back teeth (behind fold in palate) making a "tut-tut" or "tsk" sound. Repeat for 1 minute.

2. Move your tongue around, keeping it at the top of your palate, and then move it toward the back of your mouth as far as it will go. Hold the tip of your tongue at the back of your palate for 1 minute.

3. With your tongue, hold a spoon or Popsicle stick at the top of your mouth. Push upward, keeping it tight against the roof of your mouth. Hold it there for at least 1 minute, longer if you can.

Day 22

Breakfast:

BLUEBERRY CHIA PUDDING

Serves 1

Ingredients

2 cups milk or coconut milk

½ cup chia seeds

2 tablespoons coconut oil

½ teaspoon cinnamon

½ cup blueberries

Directions

Combine all ingredients in a blender. Serve cold.

Lunch: Roasted pepitas, pumpkin, and quinoa salad with feta cheese and olive oil.

Dinner: Pan-fried cabbage and bacon served in chicken or beef broth.

Day 23

Breakfast: Skip.

Lunch: Fresh mint scrambled eggs cooked in cream with chopped zucchini.

Dinner: Chicken liver stir-fry with crispy bacon and assorted greens, served with kombucha.

Day 24

Breakfast: Soft poached eggs with pan-fried tomatoes and kefir.

Lunch: Pan-fried haloumi cheese with walnuts, cinnamon, and chopped apple.

Dinner:

TURKEY CUCUMBER ROLLS

Serves 2 to 3

Equipment

Toothpicks

Ingredients

3 tablespoons cream cheese

2 jalapeños, chopped

1 bunch cilantro

Sea salt

2 whole cucumbers, peeled

½ pound ground oven-baked turkey

1 carrot, shredded

1 onion, finely chopped

Directions

1. Use blender to combine cream cheese, jalapeños, cilantro, and salt. Place in a bowl.

2. With a vegetable peeler, slice cucumbers lengthwise into long, thin strips. Lay flat, side by side, on parchment paper.

3. Spread cream cheese mixture over cucumber slices.

4. Layer turkey on top.

5. Add carrot and onion to one of the cucumber slices in a narrow line next to the turkey.

6. Roll parchment paper lengthwise to create one long roll of cucumber strips. Slice the cucumber strips into smaller, separate rolls.

7. Insert toothpicks into separate rolls and serve.

Day 25

Breakfast: Skip.

Lunch:

AVOCADO CAULIFLOWER TABBOULEH

Serves 2

Ingredients

1 medium head cauliflower, cored and roughly chopped

6 green onions, chopped

2 large tomatoes, seeded and chopped

1 cucumber, seeded and chopped

1 large bunch flat-leaf parsley, roughly chopped

1 large handful mint leaves, roughly chopped

Juice of 2 lemons

¼ cup extra-virgin olive oil

1 teaspoon sea salt

1 teaspoon black pepper

½ eggplant, chopped

1 avocado, chopped

Directions

1. In a food processor pulse the cauliflower until it's broken into small, grain-size pieces. Remove from food processor and set aside.

2. Pulse onions, tomatoes, cucumber, parsley, and mint separately. Once a light, fluffy consistency is achieved, transfer the mixture to a mixing bowl and combine with cauliflower.

3. Add lemon juice, olive oil, salt, and pepper to taste.

4. Fry eggplant until brown and serve with cauliflower tabbouleh and chopped avocado.

Dinner:

TURMERIC CHICKEN THIGHS

Serves 2

Ingredients

1 tablespoon extra-virgin olive oil

1 ½ teaspoons turmeric

3 or 4 chicken thighs

2 to 3 tablespoons butter

3 to 4 cloves garlic, chopped

1 bunch fresh rosemary

1 cup spinach

1 teaspoon sea salt

1 teaspoon black pepper

Directions

1. Preheat oven to 400°F.

2. Combine olive oil and tumeric in a bowl. Coat chicken with this mixture and place in a baking pan.

3. Cover with half of butter, then add garlic and rosemary. Bake for 30 to 35 minutes until brown.

4. While the chicken is cooking, heat remaining butter in pan. Add spinach and cook until soft.

5. Spice to taste. Serve chicken and spinach with juices from the baking pan.

Day 26

Breakfast: Mashed avocado with turmeric eggs and mushrooms.

Lunch: Liver pâté and hard cheese platter.

Dinner:

WHOLE FISH WITH HAZELNUT, CARROT, AND ONION STUFFING

Serves 2

Ingredients

1 onion, chopped

1 carrot, chopped

2 tablespoons ghee or other animal fat

2 ounces hazelnuts, chopped

1 bunch parsley, chopped

1 egg

Juice of 1 lemon

1 whole sea bass or snapper

1 tablespoon olive oil

Directions

1. Preheat oven to 375°F.

2. Fry onion and carrot in ghee until soft.

3. Add hazelnuts and parsley; toss and cook for 2 minutes, until brown.

4. Add egg and sauté until mixture is cooked through.

4. Top with lemon juice.

5. Place inside whole fish (gutted), drizzle olive oil over fish, and bake for 20 to 30 minutes or until fish is crispy or flakes easily.

Day 27

Breakfast: Skip.

Lunch: Chickpea, radish, and cabbage salad, served with a glass of kefir on the side.

Dinner: Pan-fried steak served with garlic butter and broccoli.

Day 28

Breakfast: Plantains and basil fried in duck fat, served with walnuts.

Lunch: Salad of leafy greens, pumpkin seeds, walnuts, and parmesan cheese, dressed with olive oil.

Dinner: Oven-baked chicken thighs with lentils, oregano, chopped carrot, zucchini, and onions.

WEEK 5: REINTRODUCING RESTAURANT FOODS

In the first four weeks, you've learned to completely remove packaged foods from your diet and how to cook fast, tasty, and nourishing meals in your own kitchen. However, the reality of modern life is that it's very difficult to cook all of your meals. In Week 5, you'll learn to reincorporate restaurant foods in moderation.

Stick to the 80/20 rule: Four out of every five meals should be made at home.

When you *do* eat out, make sure to ask your server which oils and sweeteners are used to prepare the food. Align your order as closely as possible to the principles we've discussed. Usually this will mean going with meals that don't have sauces or ordering simply prepared meals or salads.

You want to have no more than 9 teaspoons of added sugar per day. If you do have a dessert or sweet snack, avoid added sugar for the next two days.

Before you eat: Voice Exercise
(once before each meal)

Exercise your voice and throat muscles by humming.

Close your eyes and take a deep breath into your diaphragm for three seconds. Then let out a quiet hum—it should be deep, but everyone's will be different. Picture the hum starting in your stomach and moving like a violin bow over your vocal cords. Do this for two minutes.

Then touch your tongue to your palate. You should notice the hum getting slightly higher, and your upper jaw should vibrate. Hum into your upper jaw like that for another two minutes.

Day 29

Breakfast: Homemade granola with yogurt.

Lunch: Green basil pesto eggs (see page 204 for the pesto recipe.)

Dinner:

BUTTERY CHILI BEEF BOWL

Serves 4

Ingredients

1 onion, chopped

1 red bell pepper, chopped

1 to 2 tablespoons coconut oil or lard

2 to 3 cups ground beef

2 teaspoons salt

3 tablespoons ghee or butter

2 tomatoes, chopped

2 stalks celery, chopped

1 to 2 red chili peppers, chopped

¼ cup tomato paste

1 ½ teaspoons cumin

1 cup water

10 ounces cheddar cheese, shredded

Directions

1. Cook onions and pepper in a large pan with coconut oil on medium to high heat until slightly brown.

2. Add beef and salt.

3. Add ghee, tomatoes, celery, chilies, tomato paste, cumin, and 1 cup water to the pan.

4. Bring to a boil, then reduce heat to low-medium and simmer for 1 to 2 hours, stirring every 30 minutes or so.

5. Serve in large bowl with cheddar sprinkled on top.

Day 30

Breakfast: Skip.

Lunch:

AVOCADO SOUP

Serves 2

Ingredients

1 tablespoon ghee or butter	2 cups cream
4 cups beef or chicken broth	1 teaspoon lime juice
2 ripe avocados, peeled and mashed	¼ teaspoon ground cumin
½ cup onion, finely chopped	Salt and pepper
1 clove garlic	1 bunch fresh cilantro

Directions

1. Heat ghee in a pot on medium heat.

2. Add broth, avocados, onion, garlic, cream, and lime juice and bring to a boil.

3. If desired, transfer to a blender and process to make smooth, then return to pot. Add cumin, salt, and pepper. *Note:* Blending hot soup can cause an explosion. To avoid an explosion, be sure to remove the cap or stopper from the blender, and fill the blender no more than halfway. Place the lid on the blender and cover the hole with a thick tea towel. Hold the towel and start the blender on low.

4. Cook on medium heat for 5 minutes, then transfer to a serving bowl and top with fresh cilantro.

5. Serve with kombucha.

Dinner: Pan-fried salmon in miso paste with kale and spring onions.

Day 31

Breakfast: Boiled egg platter with hummus and celery sticks.

Lunch: Tuna, olive oil, and baby spinach salad with chili dressing, served with sauerkraut.

Dinner:

OVEN-BAKED CHICKEN LEGS WITH SWEET POTATO CHIPS

Serves 4

Ingredients

½ cup olive oil

Sea salt

Pepper

2 to 3 cloves garlic, chopped

6 to 8 chicken drumsticks

1 sweet potato, sliced

1 bunch fresh rosemary, chopped

7 ounces fresh watercress

Directions

1. Preheat oven to 375°F.

2. Combine ¼ cup olive oil and the salt, pepper, and garlic in a bowl. Glaze chicken with mixture.

3. Coat a baking pan with 1 tablespoon olive oil. Place sweet potato on the pan. Top with a light coating of olive oil, leaving a small amount to reglaze. Place chicken on top of sweet potato.

4. Bake for 20 minutes until chicken is browned.

5. Remove from oven, turn the chicken, and reglaze the chicken and sweet potato with remaining olive oil. Add rosemary.

6. Bake for another half hour until chicken is cooked through. Garnish with watercress.

Day 32

Breakfast: Skip.

Lunch: Turmeric scrambled eggs cooked with cabbage and red peppers.

Dinner:

ASIAN-STYLE SEAFOOD SOUP WITH ZUCCHINI AND CARROT NOODLES

Serves 4

Ingredients

½ pound beef, sliced thin

Coconut oil or lard

2 carrots

4 medium zucchini

2 cups broth (or collagen powder added to water)

2 cloves garlic, minced

¼ teaspoon ginger (minced)

2 cups bean sprouts

¼ cup chopped scallions (optional)

1 egg, soft-boiled

2 tablespoons oyster sauce

2 tablespoons apple cider vinegar

Salt

Pepper

Directions

1. In a pan, sear beef slices in coconut oil and set aside.

2. Use vegetable peeler to create thin ribbons of carrot and zucchini.

3. Combine broth, garlic, and ginger in a large pot and bring to a boil.

4. Add the carrot ribbons, bean sprouts, and scallions to the broth. Cook for about 5 minutes.

5. Add the zucchini and carrot strips and cook until soft.

6. Add beef, egg, oyster sauce, and apple cider vinegar to the soup, and season with salt and pepper to taste. Serve hot.

Day 33

Breakfast: Berry-topped yogurt with coconut oil, cinnamon, and cardamom sprinkle.

Lunch: Grilled lemon–pepper fish with onions and carrot sticks.

Dinner: Liverwurst with chicken or beef broth (pages 209 and 210), oven-baked broccoli, and potatoes.
Note: Liverwurst can be found at most supermarkets or butchers.

Day 34

Breakfast: Skip.

Lunch: Green spinach scrambled eggs.

Dinner:

PEA SOUP

Serves 2

Ingredients

2 tablespoons coconut oil or animal fat

1 onion, chopped

3 cloves garlic, minced

2 sprigs thyme, chopped

3 cups beef or chicken broth

1 cup fresh English peas

1 tablespoon apple cider vinegar

Salt and pepper

1 bunch parsley, chopped

Directions

1. Heat coconut oil in a saucepan over medium heat. Add onion, garlic, and thyme and cook for 5 minutes.

2. Add broth, peas, vinegar, salt, and pepper. Bring to a boil.

3. Reduce heat to low, add parsley, cover, and cook for 5 to 10 minutes.

4. Remove from heat and serve warm.

Day 35
Breakfast:

CREAMY GREEN COLLAGEN SMOOTHIE

Serves 1

Ingredients

2 cups spinach

½ avocado

½ banana

1 tablespoon coconut oil

2 tablespoons cream

2 tablespoon chia seeds

2 tablespoon flaxseed

1 tablespoon gelatin powder

Directions

Add all ingredients to a blender and pulse until it reaches a creamy, smooth texture.

Lunch: Mixed green leaf and herb salad with watercress, cabbage, parsley, and basil.

Dinner:

LEMONGRASS AND GINGER BAKED FISH WITH BROTH AND CUCUMBER RICE

Serves 2 to 3

Ingredients

1 whole snapper or other fish

1 cucumber, chopped

½ cup extra virgin olive oil

1 stalk fresh ginger

1 stalk lemongrass

Zest of 1 lemon

1 lime

1 bunch cilantro

1 teaspoon chili flakes

2 chilies, seeded and sliced thin

1 teaspoon pepper

1 teaspoon sea salt

1 cup chicken or beef broth

Directions

1. Preheat oven to 200°F.

2. Place foil on work surface and place fish on top.

3. Place cucumber around fish.

4. Combine olive oil and all remaining ingredients except broth in a bowl.

5. Rub oil mixture over fish. Transfer fish and foil to baking tray and bake for 30 to 35 minutes.

6. Warm broth and serve in a bowl with the fish, or separately.

7. Spice to taste.

WEEK 6: YOUR NEW NORMAL

In the five weeks leading up to this, you've retrained your mouth and body to eat and digest the way they're designed to. Personally, after six weeks of eating this way, I knew I could never go back to eating like I did before. I always *knew* that my new diet would produce big benefits for my body. But now I *felt* it. I felt better than ever.

Week 6 represents the first week of the rest of your nutritious life. Now that you've reset your body's needs, it's okay to indulge in "non-Dental Diet foods" every now and again. But you may find that you won't have the same cravings for sugary, nutrient-poor foods that you used to. It will be easier to give your body the foods it truly needs. And your weight, skin, and mental clarity will continue to thank you for it.

**Before you eat: Moving and Breathing
(once before each meal)**

Learning to breathe through your nose while you move will help you to breathe through your nose throughout the day and night.

1. Plan a 10-minute walk.

2. Before you start, put your tongue to the roof of your mouth and take 10 deep, nasal breaths.

3. Walk at a steady pace, focusing on keeping your lips closed tight, breathing in for 3 seconds and breathing out for 4 seconds.

4. If you feel out of breath, slow down.

5. As you practice, you will get better and will be able to move faster and for longer periods.

Day 36

Breakfast: Banana and roasted nuts.

Lunch: Cheese platter with guacamole and sweet potato fries.

Dinner:

PAPRIKA AND GARLIC-SPICED CHICKEN WINGS WITH ZUCCHINI FRIES

Serves 4

Ingredients

2 whole zucchini, sliced

3 tablespoons butter, melted

Sea salt

1 tablespoon paprika

4 cloves garlic, crushed

Pepper

2 pounds chicken wings

½ cup sour cream

Directions

1. Preheat oven to 375°F.

2. Add zucchini to base of roasting pan and top with butter and salt.

3. Combine paprika, garlic, and pepper in a bowl. Season chicken wings with this mixture, then add them to the roasting pan.

4. Bake for 30 minutes, until chicken is cooked through.

5. Serve warm, with sour cream on the side.

Day 37

Breakfast: Skip.

Lunch: Baked eggplant slices with oregano-spiced tomatoes and mushrooms, topped with feta cheese and olive oil.

Dinner:

SPICY PUMPKIN SOUP

Serves 2

Ingredients

2 tablespoons coconut oil, ghee, or lard

1 medium yellow onion, chopped

2 carrots, chopped

2 chili peppers, chopped

2 cups beef or chicken broth

1 butternut pumpkin, chopped

2 to 3 sage leaves

1 medium apple, cored and chopped

⅔ cup coconut milk

2 teaspoons lime juice, or to taste

Sea salt to taste

Directions

1. In a large saucepan, heat coconut oil over medium heat and add onion, carrots, and chilies. Sauté until brown and soft.

2. Add broth, pumpkin, and sage leaves. Simmer for 15 to 20 minutes, then remove sage leaves.

3. Add the remaining ingredients. Heat gently and adjust seasonings to taste.

Day 38

Breakfast: Eggs served on buttered cauliflower rice

Lunch: Pan-fried asparagus, served with carrot chips baked in coconut oil

Dinner:

CHILI-BUTTER PRAWN SALAD

Serves 2

Ingredients

3 tablespoons butter, melted	2 avocados, cubed
1 bunch parsley, chopped	1 pound prawns, cooked
1 red chili, chopped	Juice of 2 limes
1 teaspoon turmeric	Sea salt
1 mango, cubed	1 head lettuce

Directions

1. Combine butter, parsley, and chili in a bowl. Add turmeric. Mix until consistent.

2. Add mango and avocados to a large bowl with prawns and mix well.

3. Pour butter mixture over salad and toss. Squeeze lime juice in, and add sea salt to taste. Serve on lettuce.

Day 39

Breakfast: Sliced and pan-fried pear and walnut salad served with yogurt

Lunch:

ROASTED POTATO SKINS WITH SOUR CREAM DIP

Serves 1 to 2

Ingredients

4 large potatoes, baked

4 tablespoons butter, melted

1 onion, diced

2 cups (8 ounces) cheddar cheese, shredded

4 cloves garlic, crushed

1 bunch fresh parsley, chopped

8 slices bacon

1 tablespoon Parmesan cheese, grated

½ teaspoon salt

⅛ teaspoon pepper

½ cup sour cream

Directions

1. Preheat oven to 475°F.

2. Cut potatoes in half and scoop out pulp, leaving skins intact. Place skins on baking pan.

3. Combine butter with onion, cheddar cheese, garlic, and parsley and fill potato skins.

4. Bake for 8 minutes, then turn over to bake for another 10 minutes.

5. Fry bacon in pan until crisp, then cut into small squares.

6. Sprinkle bacon on top of filled potato skins, along with Parmesan cheese.

7. Season with salt and pepper, and serve with sour cream.

Dinner: Liver, onion, and bacon stir-fry with turmeric and fresh basil.

Day 40

Breakfast: Fried eggs and haloumi cheese with sauerkraut.

Lunch:

TURMERIC CHICKEN CABBAGE ROLLS

Serves 2 to 3

Ingredients

1 cabbage	Salt
1 pound ground chicken	Pepper
1 onion, chopped	½ cup tomato paste
1 egg	2 to 3 tablespoons coconut oil or lard
1 tablespoon turmeric	1 cup water

Directions

1. In a shallow pan, bring salted water to a boil. Separate 6 to 8 cabbage leaves and cook for 2 to 4 minutes, until softened.

2. Add chicken, onion, egg, turmeric, salt and pepper to taste, and tomato paste to bowl and mix.

3. Add some of the chicken mixture to the center of each cabbage leaf, roll tightly, and secure with toothpicks (optional).

4. Add coconut oil or lard to pan. Place cabbage rolls in a pan or skillet, and add 1 cup of water. Bring to a boil, then reduce heat to low and simmer for 40 minutes. Stir and baste cabbage every 10 minutes.

5. Serve warm.

Dinner: Pan-fried steak served with crushed almonds, blue cheese, and broccoli.

Day 41
Breakfast: Skip.

Lunch: Avocado, fennel, and parsley salad with olive oil dressing.

Dinner: Baked salmon filet with carrots and baby tomato.

Day 42
Breakfast: Scrambled eggs with asparagus and cream.

Lunch: Green bean and lentil salad with feta cheese.

Dinner:

MUSHROOM MASALA BAKE

Serves 4

Ingredients
Coconut oil or lard

3 stalks celery, chopped

1 onion, chopped

¾ pound wild mushrooms, chopped

1 head broccoli, chopped

4 eggs, beaten

1 cup broth

¼ cup milk

1 cup heavy cream

4 tablespoons butter

1 tablespoon cardamom

1 tablespoon turmeric

1 tablespoon dry cloves

2 cups shredded Gouda cheese

Directions

1. Preheat oven to 350°F.

2. Heat coconut oil in a pan. Add celery and onion and cook until soft.

3. Add mushrooms and broccoli to pan, and stir until soft and brown.

4. Add eggs and stir in evenly. Add broth, stir until eggs are cooked, then remove from heat and set aside.

5. In a small bowl, mix milk, cream, butter, cardamom, turmeric, and cloves.

6. Add mushroom mixture and seasoned milk to a baking tray. Sprinkle cheese over the top.

7. Cover with foil and bake for 30 minutes. Remove foil and bake for 40 more minutes until topping is golden and crisp.

8. Serve warm.

CONCLUSION

A FUTURE OF SMILING

I share *The Dental Diet* with you with great pride. I hope that it inspires you, like Price's work inspired me, and deepens your appreciation for food.

The concepts we've explored in this book are both very old and very new. But the reality is that we are at the very beginnings of our understanding of the relationship between our bodies and nutrition. Evolutionary science, mineral balance, the microbiome, and epigenetics are all fields that are only now starting to bloom.

Our bodies are an intricate reflection of our ancestral health, the microbes that live within us, and our genes. Epigenetics has taught us that our reflection is more malleable than we used to think. Every piece of food we eat sends a specific message to our ever-listening genes and sparks a chain reaction that starts in our mouth and travels throughout our entire body.

One of the most important things we've recently learned about this system is how much it depends on a balance of fat-soluble vitamins, calcium, and pre- and probiotics to be in tip-top shape.

While there is still much to learn, we have to realize that our body has natural healing powers that can help keep us out of the dentist's chair or the doctor's office. But our body needs the right fuel to activate those powers. Our diet is of infinite importance to our health.

I hope this book gives you a sense of power—the power not just to *maintain* your mouth and teeth, but to strengthen your teeth and make them healthier *than ever.*

You may think, *Hang on; you didn't mention this mineral, or this vitamin, or this condition.* The Dental Diet works under the principle that your mouth is the baseline for your health. When you consume the nutrients from foods that manage your dental health, the rest falls into place.

People with deeper chronic conditions may need to undergo a deeper dietary analysis to see what their body is missing. But they should *first* work with the principles that establish good oral health.

While sugar and processed foods and erratic brushing are all obstacles to dental health, they're really symptoms of a much more basic obstacle: a feeling of helplessness when it comes to our mouths.

For many of us, that feeling has been ingrained since we were little. We were taught to brush our teeth every morning and night, and we were told sugar might rot our teeth, but that was essentially the sum total of our dental education. Even if we brushed and flossed, generally stayed away from sugar, and saw the dentist regularly, it didn't guarantee healthy teeth. We still had to have cavities filled and our wisdom teeth pulled out. We might have undergone root canals, not to mention the extensive orthodontic treatments many of us had to endure when we were young.

It all added up to the sense that, no matter what we did, our mouths and teeth were inevitably going to have problems, and the best we could do was to patch them up when they arose. People who didn't have cavities or didn't need braces were just lucky. They had "good teeth." Either you were born that way or you weren't, and that's all there was to it.

I hope I've shown you that there's so much more to it. You *do* have control over the health and well-being of your mouth, teeth, and entire body. And that power lies in what you eat.

To be sure, avoiding certain foods is important. (I've made several cases against refined sugar, carbohydrates, and processed food in this book for a reason.) But knowing what we can't do doesn't give us a sense of power. It might even contribute to a sense of helplessness. After all, while we were always told to avoid too much sugar, we were never really told what we could replace it with, were we?

That's the crux of it. It's knowing what we *can* do that empowers us. That's why the Dental Diet is more about adding the right foods and nutrients to your plate than it is about taking foods off it.

When my patients walk out of my office armed with the knowledge that they can do something truly proactive about their dental health, they have a very different look on their face than they had coming in. They have confidence and peace of mind. If you follow the plan outlined in *The Dental Diet*, you'll have them yourself and be proud to show off your new and improved smile.

Practice makes perfect, and following the Dental Diet will become a little bit easier every day. As you become more thoughtful about what you eat and where it's from, the foods that taste good to you will change. Your taste buds will awaken from their sugar coma. Before you know it, eating natural, nutrient-rich foods will become second nature and you'll start feeling better due to eating this way. Your teeth will feel great and your mouth will feel great. You'll spend less time at each dental appointment and need less treatment.

Of course, the benefits won't stop at your mouth. Digestive issues you have will begin to clear up. You'll gravitate to a healthier weight. You'll have more energy. Your mind will become clearer. In short, your mouth, body, and mind will start functioning as they were designed to.

It's all up to you now. No longer can you say that you're powerless or that you just don't have "good teeth." The answers to dental problems are in our food. It's as simple as that.

So dig in! I hope you enjoy your journey to strong teeth and a long, healthy life. Along the way, I think you'll come to see what humans have forgotten over the years: that food is truly the best medicine.

REFERENCES

Chapter 1

1. Peterson, Poul Erik. "Challenges to improvement of oral health in the 21st century-the approach of the WHO Global Oral Health Prgramme." *International dental journal 54, no. S6 (2004): 329–343.*

2. National Institutes of Health. "Dental caries (tooth decay) in children (age 2 to 11)." U.S. Department of Health and Human Services, 2014. Web. 13 Dec. 2016. <http://www.nidcr.nih.gov/DataStatistics/FindDataByTopic/ DentalCaries/DentalCariesChildren2to11.htm>.

3. Templeton, Sarah-Kate. "Rotten Teeth Put 26,000 Chilrdren in Hospital." *The Times & The Sunday Times,* July 13, 2014. www.thetimes.co.uk/article/rotten- teeth-put-26000-children-in-hospital-br5zzzpnfz0. Accessed 13 May 2016.

4. Thomsen, Michael. "Braces, Pointless and Essential." *The Atlantic.* Atlantic Media Company, 9 July 2015. Web. https://www.theatlantic.com/health/ archive/2015/07/braces-dentures-history/397934/. Accessed 26 May 2016.

5. Mascarelli, Amanda Leigh. "Braces are for grown-ups too." *Los Angeles Times.* 4 July 2011. Web. 13 Dec. 2016. <http://articles.latimes.com/2011/jul/04/ health/la-he-adult-braces-20110704>.

6. Friedman, Jay W. "The prophylactic extraction of third molars: a public health hazard." *American journal of public health* 97, no. 9 (2007): 1554–1559.

7. "Dentists in the US: market research report." *Ibisworld.* 2016. Web. 13 Dec. 2016. http://www.ibisworld.com/industry/default.aspx?indid=1557.

8. Forshaw, R. J. "Dental health and disease in ancient Egypt." *British dental journal* 206, no. 8 (2009): 421–424.

9. Gibbons, A. "An evolutionary theory of dentistry." *Science* 336.6084 (2012): 973–975.

10. Corruccini, Robert S. "Australian aboriginal tooth succession, interproximal attrition, and Begg's theory." *American journal of orthodontics and dentofacial orthopedics* 97, no. 4 (1990): 349–357.

11. Corruccini, Robert S. "An epidemiologic transition in dental occlusion in world populations." *American journal of orthodontics* 86, no. 5 (1984): 419–426.

12. Solow, Beni, and Liselotte Sonnesen. "Head posture and malocclusions." *European journal of orthodontics* 20, no. 6 (1998): 685–693.

13. Centers for Disease Control and Prevention. "National diabetes statistics report: estimates of diabetes and its burden in the United States, 2014." Atlanta, Georgia: U.S. Department of Health and Human services, 2014.

14. Rysdal, Kai. "Processed Foods Make Up 70 Percent of the U.S. Diet." *Marketplace,* 12 Mar. 2013, Web. <www.marketplace.org/2013/03/12/life/big-book/ processed-foods-make-70-percent-us-diet>. Accessed 5 May 2016.

15. Powell, Nick, Benedict Huntley, Thomas Beech, William Knight, Hannah Knight, and Christopher J. Corrigan. "Increased prevalence of gastrointestinal symptoms in patients with allergic disease." *Postgraduate medical journal* 83, no. 977 (2007): 182–186.

16. Cooper, Glinda S., Milele L. K. Bynum, and Emily C. Somers. "Recent insights in the epidemiology of autoimmune diseases: improved prevalence estimates and understanding of clustering of diseases." *Journal of autoimmunity* 33, no. 3 (2009): 197–207.

17. Brown, Rebecca C., Alan H. Lockwood, and Babasaheb R. Sonawane. "Neurodegenerative diseases: an overview of environmental risk factors." *Environmental health perspectives* 113.9 (2005): 1250–1256.

Chapter 2

1. Price, A Weston. *Nutrition and Physical Degeneration*. Lemon Grove, California: Price Pottenger Foundation, 1945.

2. Ibid.

3. Ibid.

4. Ibid.

5. Ibid.

6. Rasmussen, Morten, Xiaosen Guo, Yong Wang, Kirk E. Lohmueller, Simon Rasmussen, Anders Albrechtsen, Line Skotte, et al. "An aboriginal Australian genome reveals separate human dispersals into Asia." *Science* 334, no. 6052 (2011): 94–98.

Chapter 3

1. Song, F., Susan O'Meara, P. Wilson, S. Golder, and J. Kleijnen. "The effectiveness and cost-effectiveness of prophylactic removal of wisdom teeth." *Health Technol Assess.* 4, no. 15 (2000): 1–55.

2. Friedman, Jay W. "The prophylactic extraction of third molars: a public health hazard." *American journal of public health* 97, no. 9 (2007): 1554–1559.

3. Rabin, Roni Caryn. "Wisdom of having that tooth removed," *New York Times,* 5 Sept. 2011. http://www.nytimes.com/2011/09/06/health/06consumer. html?_r=0, (accessed 25 May 2015).

4. Preuss, Todd M. "The human brain: rewired and running hot." *Annals of the New York Academy of Sciences* 1225, no. S1 (2011): E182–E191.

5. Aiello, Leslie C., and Peter Wheeler. "The expensive-tissue hypothesis: the brain and the digestive system in human and primate evolution." *Current anthropology* 36, no. 2 (1995): 199–221.

6. Price, A Weston. *Nutrition and Physical Degeneration.* Lemon Grove, California: Price Pottenger Foundation, 1945.

7. Corruccinni, Robert S., and L. Darrell Whitley. "Occlusal variation in a rural Kentucky community." *American journal of orthodontics* 79, no. 3 (1981): 250–262.

8. Corruccini, Robert S. "An epidemiologic transition in dental occlusion in world populations." *American journal of orthodontics* 86.5 (1984): 419–426.

9. Norton N. S., *Netter's head and neck anatomy for dentistry,* 3rd ed. Milton, Ontario: Elsevier/Saunders, 2012.

10. Lundberg, Jon O. "Nitric oxide and the paranasal sinuses." *Anatomical record* 291.11 (2008): 1479–1484.

11. Behbehani, Faraj, Jon Ärtun, and Lukman Thalib. "Prediction of mandibular third-molar impaction in adolescent orthodontic patients." *American journal of orthodontics and dentofacial orthopedics* 130, no. 1 (2006): 47–55.

12. Guimarães, Kátia C., Luciano F. Drager, Pedro R. Genta, Bianca F. Marcondes, and Geraldo Lorenzi-Filho. "Effects of oropharyngeal exercises on patients with moderate obstructive sleep apnea syndrome." *American journal of respiratory and critical care medicine* 179, no. 10 (2009): 962–966.

13. Patil, Susheel P., Hartmut Schneider, Alan R. Schwartz, and Philip L. Smith. "Adult obstructive sleep apnea: pathophysiology and diagnosis." *Chest journal* 132, no. 1 (2007): 325–337.

14. Samuels, Curtis A., George Butterworth, Tony Roberts, Lida Graupner, and Graham Hole. "Facial aesthetics: babies prefer attractiveness to symmetry." *Perception* 23, no. 7 (1994): 823–831.

15. Peres, Karen Glazer, Andreia Morales Cascaes, Marco Aurelio Peres, Flavio Fernando Demarco, Iná Silva Santos, Alicia Matijasevich, and Aluisio J. D. Barros. "Exclusive breastfeeding and risk of dental malocclusion." *Pediatrics* 136, no. 1 (2015): e60–e67.

16. Boyd, K., et al. "Human malocclusion and changed feeding practices since the Industrial Revolution." Presented at the International Society for Evolution, Medicine & Public Health Annual Meeting 2015.

17. Enlow, Donald H., and Mark G. Hans. *Essentials of facial growth*. Philadelphia: Saunders, 1996.

18. Gungor, Ahmet Yalcin, and Hakan Turkkahraman. "Effects of airway problems on maxillary growth: a review."*European journal of dentistry* 3, no. 3 (2009): 250.

19. Holmberg, Hans, and Sten Linder-Aronson. "Cephalometric radiographs as a means of evaluating the capacity of the nasal and nasopharyngeal airway." *American journal of orthodontics* 76, no. 5 (1979): 479–490.

20. Hu, Zhiai, et al. "The effect of teeth extraction for orthodontic treatment on the upper airway: a systematic review." *Sleep and breathing* 19.2 (2015): 441–451.

21. Mew, John. "Facial changes in identical twins treated by different orthodontic techniques." *World journal of orthodontics* 8, no. 2 (2007): 174.

22. He, Junyun, Hung Hsuchou, Yi He, Abba J. Kastin, Yuping Wang, and Weihong Pan. "Sleep restriction impairs blood–brain barrier function." *Journal of neuroscience* 34, no. 44 (2014): 14697–14706.

23. Ting, Leon, and Atul Malhotra. "Disorders of sleep: an overview." *Primary care* 32.2 (2005): 305.

24. Eckert, Danny J., et al. "Central sleep apnea: pathophysiology and treatment." *Chest journal* 131.2 (2007): 595–607.

25. Macey, Paul M., Rajesh Kumar, Jennifer A. Ogren, Mary A. Woo, and Ronald M. Harper. "Global brain blood-oxygen level responses to autonomic challenges in obstructive sleep apnea." *PloS one* 9, no. 8 (2014): e105261.

26. "Extent and health consequences of chronic sleep loss and sleep disorders." Ch. 3 in Institute of Medicine (U.S.) Committee on Sleep Medicine and Research; Colten, H. R., and B. M. Altevogt, editors. *Sleep disorders and sleep deprivation: an unmet public health problem*. Washington, D.C.: National Academies Press, 2006.

27. Punjabi, Naresh M. "The epidemiology of adult obstructive sleep apnea." *Proceedings of the American Thoracic Society* 5, no. 2 (2008): 136–143.

28. Macey, Paul M., et al. "Brain structural changes in obstructive sleep apnea." *Sleep* 31.7 (2008): 967.

29. Kumar, Rajesh, et al. "Altered global and regional brain mean diffusivity in patients with obstructive sleep apnea." *Journal of neuroscience research* 90.10 (2012): 2043–2052.

30. Guilleminault, Christian, et al. "A cause of excessive daytime sleepiness: the upper airway resistance syndrome." *Chest* 104.3 (1993): 781–787.

31. Park, Y. Steven. "Upper airway resistance syndrome." Doctor Steven Y. Park MD (New York, NY) Integrative Solutions for Obstructive Sleep Apnea, Upper Airway Resistance Syndrome and Snoring. N.p., July 2016. http://doctorstevenpark.com/sleep-apnea-basics/upper-airway-resistance-syndrome (accessed July 2016).

32. de Godoy, Luciana B. M., et al. "Treatment of upper airway resistance syndrome in adults: Where do we stand?" *Sleep science* 8.1 (2015): 42–48.

33. Guilleminault, Christian, John L. Faul, and Riccardo Stoohs. "Sleep-disordered breathing and hypotension." *American journal of respiratory and critical care medicine* 164, no. 7 (2001): 1242–1247.

34. Kunter, Erdogan, Ozkan Yetkin, and Hakan Gunen. "UARS presenting with the symptoms of anxiety and depression." *Central European journal of medicine* 5.6 (2010): 712–715.

35. de Godoy, Luciana Balester Mello, Gabriela Pontes Luz, Luciana Oliveira Palombini, Luciana Oliveira e Silva, Wilson Hoshino, Thais Moura Guimaraes, Sergio Tufik, Lia Bittencourt, and Sonia Maria Togeiro. "Upper Airway Resistance Syndrome Patients Have Worse Sleep Quality Compared to Mild Obstructive Sleep Apnea." *PLoS ONE* 11, no. 5 (2016): e0156244–e0156244.

36. El Shakankiry, Hanan M. "Sleep physiology and sleep disorders in childhood." *Nature and science of sleep* 3 (2011): 101.

37. Gozal, David. "Obstructive sleep apnea in children: implications for the developing central nervous system." *Seminars in pediatric neurology* 15, no. 2. W. B. Saunders, 2008.

38. Scott, Nicola, et al. "Sleep patterns in children with ADHD: a population-based cohort study from birth to 11 years." *Journal of sleep research* 22.2 (2013): 121–128.

39. Iftikhar, Imran H., Christopher E. Kline, and Shawn D. Youngstedt. "Effects of exercise training on sleep apnea: a meta-analysis." *Lung* 192.1 (2014): 175–184.

40. Puhan, Milo A., et al. "Didgeridoo playing as alternative treatment for obstructive sleep apnoea syndrome: randomised controlled trial." *BMJ* 332.7536 (2006): 266–270.

Chapter 4

1. Farges, Jean-Christophe, Aurélie Bellanger, Maxime Ducret, Elisabeth Aubert-Foucher, Béatrice Richard, Brigitte Alliot-Licht, Françoise Bleicher, and Florence Carrouel. "Human odontoblast-like cells produce nitric oxide with antibacterial activity upon TLR2 activation." *Frontiers in physiology* 6, June (2015): 185.

2. Hu, B., et al. "Bone marrow cells can give rise to ameloblast-like cells." *Journal of dental research* 85.5 (2006): 416–421.

3. Takayanagi, Hiroshi. "Osteoimmunology: shared mechanisms and crosstalk between the immune and bone systems." *Nature reviews immunology* 7.4 (2007): 292–304.

4. Arana-Chavez, Victor E., and Luciana F. Massa. "Odontoblasts: the cells forming and maintaining dentine." *International journal of biochemistry & cell biology* 36, no. 8 (2004): 1367–1373.

5. Nagaoka, Shigetaka, Youichi Miyazaki, Hong-Jih Liu, Yuko Iwamoto, Motoo Kitano, and Masataka Kawagoe. "Bacterial invasion into dentinal tubules of human vital and nonvital teeth." *Journal of endodontics* 21, no. 2 (1995): 70–73.

6. Berdal, A., P. Papagerakis, D. Hotton, I. Bailleul-Forestier, and J. L. Davideau. "Ameloblasts and odontoblasts, target-cells for 1, 25-dihydroxyvitamin D3: a review." *International journal of developmental biology* 39, no. 1 (2003): 257–262.

7. Lemire, Jacques M., J. S. Adams, R. Sakai, and S. C. Jordan. "1 alpha, 25-dihydroxyvitamin D3 suppresses proliferation and immunoglobulin production by normal human peripheral blood mononuclear cells." *Journal of clinical investigation* 74, no. 2 (1984): 657.

8. Tang, Jun, Ru Zhou, Dror Luger, Wei Zhu, Phyllis B. Silver, Rafael S. Grajewski, Shao-Bo Su, Chi-Chao Chan, Luciano Adorini, and Rachel R. Caspi. "Calcitriol suppresses antiretinal autoimmunity through inhibitory effects on the Th17 effector response." *Journal of immunology* 182, no. 8 (2009): 4624–4632.

9. Papagerakis, P., M. MacDougall, D. Hotton, I. Bailleul-Forestier, M. Oboeuf, and A. Berdal. "Expression of amelogenin in odontoblasts." *Bone* 32, no. 3 (2003): 228–240.

10. Schroth, R. J., R. Rabbani, G. Loewen, and M. E. Moffatt. "Vitamin D and dental caries in children." *Journal of dental research* 95, no. 2 (2016): 173–179.

11. Hildebolt, Charles F. "Effect of vitamin D and calcium on periodontitis." *Journal of periodontology* 76, no. 9 (2005): 1576–1587.

12. Heaney, Robert P. "Vitamin D and calcium interactions: functional outcomes." *American journal of clinical nutrition* 88, no. 2 (2008): 541S–544S.

13. Guimarães, Gustavo Narvaes, Thaisângela Lopes Rodrigues, Ana Paula de Souza, Sergio Roberto Line, and Marcelo Rocha Marques. "Parathyroid hormone (1–34) modulates odontoblast proliferation and apoptosis via PKA and PKC-dependent pathways." *Calcified tissue international* 95, no. 3 (2014): 275–281.

14. Ramagopalan, Sreeram V., Andreas Heger, Antonio J. Berlanga, Narelle J. Maugeri, Matthew R. Lincoln, Amy Burrell, Lahiru Handunnetthi, et al. "A ChIP-seq defined genome-wide map of vitamin D receptor binding: associations with disease and evolution." *Genome research* 20, no. 10 (2010): 1352–1360.

15. Nair, Rathish, and Arun Maseeh. "Vitamin D: the 'sunshine' vitamin." *Journal of pharmacology and pharmacotherapeutics* 3, no. 2 (2012): 118.

16. Garland, Cedric F., Frank C. Garland, Edward D. Gorham, Martin Lipkin, Harold Newmark, Sharif B. Mohr, and Michael F. Holick. "The role of vitamin D in cancer prevention." *American journal of public health* 96, no. 2 (2006): 252–261.

17. Littlejohns, Thomas J., William E. Henley, Iain A. Lang, Cedric Annweiler, Olivier Beauchet, Paulo H. M. Chaves, Linda Fried, et al. "Vitamin D and the risk of dementia and Alzheimer disease." *Neurology* 83, no. 10 (2014): 920–928.

18. Pierrot-Deseilligny, Charles, and Jean-Claude Souberbielle. "Contribution of vitamin D insufficiency to the pathogenesis of multiple sclerosis." *Therapeutic advances in neurological disorders* 6, no.2 (2013): 81–116.

19. Xu, Qun, Christine G. Parks, Lisa A. DeRoo, Richard M. Cawthon, Dale P. Sandler, and Honglei Chen. "Multivitamin use and telomere length in women." *American journal of clinical* 89 (2009): 1857–63.

20. Vimaleswaran, Karani S., Diane J. Berry, Chen Lu, Emmi Tikkanen, Stefan Pilz, Linda T. Hiraki, Jason D. Cooper, et al. "Causal relationship between obesity and vitamin D status: bi-directional Mendelian randomization analysis of multiple cohorts." *PLoS Med* 10, no. 2 (2013): 1–13.

21. Khayyat, Yasir, and Suzan Attar. "Vitamin D deficiency in patients with irritable bowel syndrome: does it exist?" *Oman medical journal* 30, no. 2 (2015): 115.

22. Tavakkoli, Anna, Daniel DiGiacomo, Peter H. Green, and Benjamin Lebwohl. "Vitamin D status and concomitant autoimmunity in celiac disease." *Journal of clinical gastroenterology* 47, no. 6 (2013): 515.

23. Blanck, Stacey, and Faten Aberra. "Vitamin D deficiency is associated with ulcerative colitis disease activity." *Digestive diseases and sciences* 58, no. 6 (2013): 1698–1702.

24. Ham, Maggie, Maria S. Longhi, Conor Lahiff, Adam Cheifetz, Simon Robson, and Alan C. Moss. "Vitamin D levels in adults with Crohn's disease are responsive to disease activity and treatment." *Inflammatory bowel diseases* 20, no. 5 (2014): 856.

25. Loeser, Richard F. "Age-related changes in the musculoskeletal system and the development of osteoarthritis." *Clinics in geriatric medicine* 26, no. 3 (2010): 371–386.

26. Bolland, Mark J., Andrew Grey, Alison Avenell, Greg D. Gamble, and Ian R. Reid. "Calcium supplements with or without vitamin D and risk of cardiovascular events: reanalysis of the Women's Health Initiative limited access dataset and meta-analysis." *BMJ* 342 (2011): d2040.

27. Semba, R., and K. Kramer. "The discovery of the vitamins." *Ann Nutr Metab* 61, no. 3 (2012): 181–270.

28. Dam, Henrik. "The antihaemorrhagic vitamin of the chick. Occurrence and chemical nature." *Nature* 135, no. 18 (1935): 652–653.

29. Howard, James Bryant, and Gary L. Nelsestuen. "Isolation and characterization of vitamin K–dependent region of bovine blood clotting factor X." *Proceedings of the National Academy of Sciences* 72, no. 4 (1975): 1281–1285.

30. Iłowiecki, Maciej. *Dzieje nauki polskiej*. Warszawa: Wydawnictwo Interpress, 1981, p. 177.

31. Hauschka, P. V. "Osteocalcin: the vitamin K–dependent Ca2+-binding protein of bone matrix." *Pathophysiology of haemostasis and thrombosis* 16, no. 3–4 (1986): 258–272.

32. Schurgers, Leon J., Ellen C. M. Cranenburg, and Cees Vermeer. "Matrix GLA-protein: the calcification inhibitor in need of vitamin K." *Thrombosis and haemostasis* 100, no. 4 (2008): 593–603.

33. Luo, Guangbin, Patricia Ducy, Marc D. McKee, Gerald J. Pinero, Evelyne Loyer, Richard R. Behringer, and Gérard Karsenty. "Spontaneous calcification of arteries and cartilage in mice lacking matrix GLA protein."*Nature* 386, no. 6620 (1997): 78–81.

34. Geleijnse, Johanna M., Cees Vermeer, Diederick E. Grobbee, Leon J. Schurgers, Marjo H. J. Knapen, Irene M. Van Der Meer, Albert Hofman, and Jacqueline C. M. Witteman. "Dietary intake of menaquinone is associated with a reduced risk of coronary heart disease: the Rotterdam study." *Journal of nutrition* 134, no. 11 (2004): 3100–3105.

35. Vermeer, Cees, Martin J. Shearer, Armin Zittermann, Caroline Bolton-Smith, Pawel Szulc, Stephen Hodges, Paul Walter, Walter Rambeck, Elisabeth Stöcklin, and Peter Weber. "Beyond deficiency." *European journal of nutrition* 43, no. 6 (2004): 325–335.

36. Falcone, Trasey D., Scott S. W. Kim, and Megan H. Cortazzo. "Vitamin K: fracture prevention and beyond." *PM&R* 3, no. 6 (2011): S82–S87.

37. Masterjohn, Chris. "On the trail of the elusive X-factor: a sixty-two-year-old mystery finally solved—Weston A. Price." *Weston A. Price*. Washington, D.C. Weston A. Price Foundation, 14 Feb. 2008. Web. 11 Dec. 2014.

38. Hauschka, P. V. "Osteocalcin: the vitamin K–dependent Ca2+-binding protein of bone matrix." *Pathophysiology of haemostasis and thrombosis* 16, no. 3–4 (1986): 258-272.

39. Schurgers, Leon J., Daniela V. Barreto, Fellype C. Barreto, Sophie Liabeuf, Cédric Renard, Elke J. Magdeleyns, Cees Vermeer, Gabriel Choukroun, and Ziad A. Massy. "The circulating inactive form of matrix GLA protein is a surrogate marker for vascular calcification in chronic kidney disease: a preliminary report." *Clinical journal of the American Society of Nephrology* 5, no. 4 (2010): 568–575.

40. Thomsen, Stine B., Camilla N. Rathcke, Bo Zerahn, and Henrik Vestergaard. "Increased levels of the calcification marker matrix GLA protein and the inflammatory markers YKL-40 and CRP in patients with type 2 diabetes and ischemic heart disease." *Cardiovascular diabetology* 9, no. 1 (2010): 1.

41. Westenfeld, Ralf, Thilo Krueger, Georg Schlieper, Ellen C. M. Cranenburg, Elke J. Magdeleyns, Stephan Heidenreich, Stefan Holzmann, et al. "Effect of vitamin K2 supplementation on functional vitamin K deficiency in hemodialysis patients: a randomized trial." *American journal of kidney diseases* 59, no. 2 (2012): 186–195.

42. Schurgers, Leon J., Daniela V. Barreto, Fellype C. Barreto, Sophie Liabeuf, Cédric Renard, Elke J. Magdeleyns, Cees Vermeer, Gabriel Choukroun, and Ziad A. Massy. "The circulating inactive form of matrix GLA protein is a surrogate marker for vascular calcification in chronic kidney disease: a preliminary report." *Clinical journal of the American Society of Nephrology* 5, no. 4 (2010): 568–575.

43. Shimamoto S., A. Tanaka, K. Tsuchida, K. Hayashi, and T. Sawa. "Serious coagulation dysfunction in a patient with gallstone-related cholecystitis successfully treated with vitamin K." *Japanese journal of anesthesiology* 65(4) (2016): 407–10 (Japanese).

44. Nimptsch, Katharina, Sabine Rohrmann, and Jakob Linseisen. "Dietary intake of vitamin K and risk of prostate cancer in the Heidelberg cohort of the European Prospective Investigation into Cancer and Nutrition (EPIC-Heidelberg)." *American Journal of clinical nutrition* 87, no. 4 (2008): 985–992.

45. Howe, Andrew M., and William S. Webster. "The warfarin embryopathy: a rat model showing maxillonasal hypoplasia and other skeletal disturbances." *Teratology* 46, no. 4 (1992): 379–390.

46. Harugop, Anil S., R. S. Mudhol, P. S. Hajare, A. I. Nargund, V. V. Metgudmath, and S. Chakrabarti. "Prevalence of nasal septal deviation in newborns and its precipitating factors: a cross-sectional study." *Indian journal of otolaryngology and head & neck surgery* 64, no. 3 (2012): 248–251.

47. Zile, Maija H. "Function of vitamin A in vertebrate embryonic development." *Journal of nutrition* 131, no. 3 (2001): 705–708.

48. Gilbert, Clare. "The eye signs of vitamin A deficiency." *Community eye health* 26, no. 84 (2013): 66.

49. Fennema, Owen. *Fennema's food chemistry.* New York, NY. CRC Press, Taylor & Francis, 2008, pp. 454–455.

50. Stephensen, Charles B. "Vitamin A, infection, and immune function." *Annual review of nutrition* 21, no. 1 (2001): 167–192.

51. Tanumihardjo, Sherry A. "Vitamin A and bone health: the balancing act." *Journal of clinical densitometry* 16, no. 4 (2013): 414–419.

52. Groenen, Pascal M. W., Iris A. L. M. van Rooij, Petronella G. M. Peer, Rob H. Gooskens, Gerhard A. Zielhuis, and Régine P. M. Steegers-Theunissen. "Marginal maternal vitamin B12 status increases the risk of offspring with spina bifida." *American journal of obstetrics and gynecology* 191, no. 1 (2004): 11–17.

53. Venkatesh, R. "Syndromes and anomalies associated with cleft." *Indian journal of plastic surgery* 42, no. 3 (2009): 51.

54. Schöne, F., H. Luedke, A. Hennig, W. Ochrimenko, P. Moeckel, and D. Geinitz. "The vitamin A activity of beta-carotene in growing pigs." *Archives of animal nutrition* 38, no. 3 (1988): 193–205.

Chapter 5

1. Kriss, Timothy C., and Vesna Martich Kriss. "History of the operating microscope: from magnifying glass to microneurosurgery." *Neurosurgery* 42, no. 4 (1998): 899–907.

2. Tan, Siang Yong, and Yvonne Tatsumura. "Alexander Fleming (1881–1955): discoverer of penicillin." *Singapore medical journal* 56, no. 7 (2015): 366.

3. Reyniers, J. A. "Germfree vertebrates: present status." *Annals of the New York Academy of Sciences* (1959) 78(1): 3.

4. Amieva, Manuel, and Richard M. Peek. "Pathobiology of *Helicobacter pylori*–induced gastric cancer." *Gastroenterology* 150, no. 1 (2016): 64–78.

5. Blaser, Martin J. "Who are we? Indigenous microbes and the ecology of human diseases." *EMBO reports* 7, no. 10 (2006): 956.

6. Ripple, William J., and Robert L. Beschta. "Wolves and the ecology of fear: can predation risk structure ecosystems?" *BioScience* 54, no. 8 (2004): 755–766.

7. Saint Louis, Catherine. "Feeling guilty about not flossing? Maybe there's no need." *New York Times*, 3 Aug. 2016. 11 Dec. 2016. <http://www.nytimes.com/2016/08/03/health/flossing-teeth-cavities.html>.

8. Kuramitsu, Howard K., and Bing-Yan Wang. "Virulence properties of cariogenic bacteria." *BMC oral health* 6, no. 1 (2006): 1.

9. Donlan, Rodney M. "Biofilms: microbial life on surfaces." *Emerg infect dis* 8, no. 9 (2002).

10. Nyvad, Bente, Wim Crielaard, Alex Mira, Nobuhiro Takahashi, and David Beighton. "Dental caries from a molecular microbiological perspective." *Caries research* 47, no. 2 (2012): 89–102.

11. Kuramitsu, Howard K., Xuesong He, Renate Lux, Maxwell H. Anderson, and Wenyuan Shi. "Interspecies interactions within oral microbial communities." *Microbiology and molecular biology reviews* 71, no. 4 (2007): 653–670.

12. Adler, Christina J., Keith Dobney, Laura S. Weyrich, John Kaidonis, Alan W. Walker, Wolfgang Haak, Corey J. A. Bradshaw, et al. "Sequencing ancient calcified dental plaque shows changes in oral microbiota with dietary shifts of the Neolithic and Industrial revolutions." *Nature genetics* 45, no. 4 (2013): 450–455.

13. Schnorr, Stephanie L., Marco Candela, Simone Rampelli, Manuela Centanni, Clarissa Consolandi, Giulia Basaglia, Silvia Turroni et al. "Gut microbiome of the Hadza hunter-gatherers." *Nature communications* 5 (2014).

14. Humphrey, Louise T., Isabelle De Groote, Jacob Morales, Nick Barton, Simon Collcutt, Christopher Bronk Ramsey, and Abdeljalil Bouzouggar. "Earliest evidence for caries and exploitation of starchy plant foods in Pleistocene hunter-gatherers from Morocco." *Proceedings of the National Academy of Sciences* 111, no. 3 (2014): 954–959.

15. Helander, Herbert F., and Lars Fändriks. "Surface area of the digestive tract—revisited." *Scandinavian journal of gastroenterology* 49, no. 6 (2014): 681–689.

16. Human Microbiome Project Consortium. "Structure, function and diversity of the healthy human microbiome." *Nature* 486, no. 7402 (2012): 207–214.

17. Sekirov, Inna, Shannon L. Russell, L. Caetano, M. Antunes, and B. Brett Finlay. "Gut microbiota in health and disease." *Physiological reviews* 90, no. 3 (2010): 859–904.

18. Neu, Josef, and Jona Rushing. "Cesarean versus vaginal delivery: long-term infant outcomes and the hygiene hypothesis." *Clinics in perinatology* 38, no. 2 (2011): 321–331.

19. Jost, Ted, Christophe Lacroix, Christian P. Braegger, Florence Rochat, and Christophe Chassard. "Vertical mother–neonate transfer of maternal gut bacteria via breastfeeding." *Environmental microbiology* 16, no. 9 (2014): 2891–2904.

20. Schuijt, T. J., T. van der Poll, and W. J. Wiersinga. "Gut microbiome and host defense interactions during critical illness." In: Annual Update in Intensive Care and Emergency Medicine 2012, pp. 29-40. Springer Berlin Heidelberg, 2012.

21. Wu, Hsin-Jung, and Eric Wu. "The role of gut microbiota in immune homeostasis and autoimmunity." *Gut microbes* 3, no. 1 (2012): 4–14.

22. Den Besten, Gijs, Karen van Eunen, Albert K. Groen, Koen Venema, Dirk-Jan Reijngoud, and Barbara M. Bakker. "The role of short-chain fatty acids in the interplay between diet, gut microbiota, and host energy metabolism." *Journal of lipid research* 54, no. 9 (2013): 2325–2340.

23. Bischoff, Stephan C., Giovanni Barbara, Wim Buurman, Theo Ockhuizen, Jörg-Dieter Schulzke, Matteo Serino, Herbert Tilg, Alastair Watson, and Jerry M. Wells. "Intestinal permeability—a new target for disease prevention and therapy." *BMC gastroenterology* 14, no. 1 (2014): 1.

24. Schnorr, Stephanie L., Marco Candela, Simone Rampelli, Manuela Centanni, Clarissa Consolandi, Giulia Basaglia, Silvia Turroni et al. "Gut microbiome of the Hadza hunter-gatherers." *Nature communications* 5 (2014).

25. King, Dana E., Arch G. Mainous, and Carol A. Lambourne. "Trends in dietary fiber intake in the United States, 1999–2008." *Journal of the Academy of Nutrition and Dietetics* 112, no. 5 (2012): 642–648.

26. Eaton, S. Boyd. "The ancestral human diet: what was it and should it be a paradigm for contemporary nutrition?" *Proceedings of the Nutrition Society* 65, no. 1 (2006): 1–6.

27. Eke, Paul I., Bruce A. Dye, Liang Wei, Gary D. Slade, Gina O. Thornton-Evans, Wenche S. Borgnakke, George W. Taylor, Roy C. Page, James D. Beck, and Robert J. Genco. "Update on prevalence of periodontitis in adults in the United States: NHANES 2009 to 2012." *Journal of periodontology* 86, no. 5 (2015): 611–622.

28. Nath, Sameera G., and Ranjith Raveendran. "Microbial dysbiosis in periodontitis." *Journal of Indian Society of Periodontology* 17, no. 4 (2013): 543.

29. Fasano, Alessio, Bernadette Baudry, David W. Pumplin, Steven S. Wasserman, Ben D. Tall, Julian M. Ketley, and J. B. Kaper. "Vibrio cholerae produces a second enterotoxin, which affects intestinal tight junctions." *Proceedings of the National Academy of Sciences* 88, no. 12 (1991): 5242–5246.

30. Francino, M. P. "Antibiotics and the human gut microbiome: Dysbioses and accumulation of resistances." *Frontiers in microbiology* 6 (2015): 1543.

31. Bischoff, Stephan C., Giovanni Barbara, Wim Buurman, Theo Ockhuizen, Jörg-Dieter Schulzke, Matteo Serino, Herbert Tilg, Alastair Watson, and Jerry M. Wells. "Intestinal permeability—a new target for disease prevention and therapy." *BMC gastroenterology* 14, no. 1 (2014): 1.

32. Perrier, C., and B. Corthesy. "Gut permeability and food allergies." *Clinical & experimental allergy* 41, no. 1 (2011): 20–28.

33. Ding, Shengli, and Pauline K. Lund. "Role of intestinal inflammation as an early event in obesity and insulin resistance." *Current opinion in clinical nutrition and metabolic care* 14, no. 4 (2011): 328.

34. Kelly, John R., Paul J. Kennedy, John F. Cryan, Timothy G. Dinan, Gerard Clarke, and Niall P. Hyland. "Breaking down the barriers: the gut microbiome, intestinal permeability and stress-related psychiatric disorders." *Frontiers in cellular neuroscience* 9 (2015): 392.

35. Campbell, Andrew W. "Autoimmunity and the Gut." *Autoimmune diseases* 2014 (2014): 152428.

36. Rook, G. A. W., and L. R. Brunet. "Microbes, immunoregulation, and the gut." *Gut* 54, no. 3 (2005): 317–320.

37. McLean, Mairi H., Dario Dieguez, Lindsey M. Miller, and Howard A. Young. "Does the microbiota play a role in the pathogenesis of autoimmune diseases?." *Gut* 64, no. 2 (2015): 332–341.

38. Lavanya, N., P. Jayanthi, Umadevi K. Rao, and K. Ranganathan. "Oral lichen planus: An update on pathogenesis and treatment." *Journal of Oral and Maxillofacial Pathology* 15, no. 2 (2011): 127.

39. Fasano, Alessio. "Zonulin and its regulation of intestinal barrier function: the biological door to inflammation, autoimmunity, and cancer." *Physiological reviews* 91, no. 1 (2011): 151–175.

40. Camilleri, Michael, and H. Gorman. "Intestinal permeability and irritable bowel syndrome." *Neurogastroenterology & Motility* 19, no. 7 (2007): 545–552.

41. Øyri, Styrk Furnes, Györgyi Múzes, and Ferenc Sipos. "Dysbiotic gut microbiome: A key element of Crohn's disease." *Comparative immunology, microbiology and infectious diseases* 43 (2015): 36–49.

42. Machiels, K., M. Joossens, J. Sabino, V. De Preter, I. Arijs, V. Eeckhaut, V. Ballet et al. "A decrease of the butyrate-producing species Roseburia hominis and Faecalibacterium prausnitzii defines dysbiosis in patients with ulcerative colitis." *Gut* 63, no. 8 (2014): 1275.

43. Goodson, J. M., D. Groppo, S. Halem, and E. Carpino. "Is obesity an oral bacterial disease?" *Journal of dental research* 88, no. 6 (2009): 519–523.

44. Kumar, P. S. (2016). "From focal sepsis to periodontal medicine: a century of exploring the role of the oral microbiome in systemic disease." *Journal of physiology*, 595 (2016): 465–476.

45. Riiser, Amund. "The human microbiome, asthma, and allergy." *Allergy, asthma & clinical immunology* 11, no. 1 (2015): 1.

46. Hartstra, Annick V., Kristien E. C. Bouter, Fredrik Bäckhed, and Max Nieuwdorp. "Insights into the role of the microbiome in obesity and type 2 diabetes." *Diabetes care* 38, no. 1 (2015): 159–165.

47. Ley, Ruth E. "Obesity and the human microbiome." *Current opinion in gastroenterology* 26, no. 1 (2010): 5–11.

48. Mayer, Emeran A., Rob Knight, Sarkis K. Mazmanian, John F. Cryan, and Kirsten Tillisch. "Gut microbes and the brain: paradigm shift in neuroscience." *Journal of neuroscience* 34, no. 46 (2014): 15490–15496.

49. Hedberg, Maria, Pamela Hasslöf, I. Sjöström, S. Twetman, and Christina Stecksén-Blicks. "Sugar fermentation in probiotic bacteria—an in vitro study." *Oral microbiology and immunology* 23, no. 6 (2008): 482–485.

50. Zarrinpar, Amir, Amandine Chaix, Shibu Yooseph, and Satchidananda Panda. "Diet and feeding pattern affect the diurnal dynamics of the gut microbiome." *Cell metabolism* 20, no. 6 (2014): 1006–1017.

51. Sapolsky, Robert M. *Why Zebras Don't Get Ulcers*, 3rd ed. New York, NY. Holt Paperbacks, August 26, 2004.

52. Stothart, Mason R., Colleen B. Bobbie, Albrecht I. Schulte-Hostedde, Rudy Boonstra, Rupert Palme, Nadia C. S. Mykytczuk, and Amy E. M. Newman. "Stress and the microbiome: linking glucocorticoids to bacterial community dynamics in wild red squirrels." *Biology letters* 12, no. 1 (2016): 20150875.

53. Voigt, Robin M., Christopher B. Forsyth, Stefan J. Green, Ece Mutlu, Phillip Engen, Martha H. Vitaterna, Fred W. Turek, and Ali Keshavarzian. "Circadian disorganization alters intestinal microbiota." *PloS one* 9, no. 5 (2014): e97500.

54. Matsumoto, Megumi, Ryo Inoue, Takamitsu Tsukahara, Kazunari Ushida, Hideyuki Chiji, Noritaka Matsubara, and Hiroshi Hara. "Voluntary running exercise alters microbiota composition and increases n-butyrate concentration in the rat cecum." *Bioscience, biotechnology, and biochemistry* 72, no. 2 (2008): 572–576.

55. Sing, David, and Charles F. Sing. "Impact of direct soil exposures from airborne dust and geophagy on human health." *International journal of environmental research and public health* 7, no. 3 (2010): 1205–1223.

56. Song, Se Jin, Christian Lauber, Elizabeth K. Costello, Catherine A. Lozupone, Gregory Humphrey, Donna Berg-Lyons, J. Gregory Caporaso, et al. "Cohabiting family members share microbiota with one another and with their dogs." *Elife* 2 (2013): e00458.

Chapter 6

1. Pottenger, F.M. Jr. *Pottenger's Cats: A Study in Nutrition*. Elaine Pottenger, editor, with Robert T. Pottenger, Jr. Lemon Grove, CA: Price-Pottenger Nutrition Foundation, 1995.

2. Harmon, Katherine. "Genome sequencing for the rest of us." *Scientific American*. 28 June 2010. Accessed 13 August 2010.

3. Steve Talbott, "Getting over the code delusion," *New Atlantis*, no. 28, Summer 2010, pp. 3–27.

4. Ibid.

5. Bentley, David R. "The human genome project—an overview." *Medicinal research reviews* 20, no. 3 (2000): 189–196.

6. Holoch, Daniel, and Danesh Moazed. "RNA-mediated epigenetic regulation of gene expression." *Nature reviews genetics* 16, no. 2 (2015): 71–84.

7. Kessels, Jana Elena, Inga Wessels, Hajo Haase, Lothar Rink, and Peter Uciechowski. "Influence of DNA-methylation on zinc homeostasis in myeloid cells: Regulation of zinc transporters and zinc binding proteins." *Journal of trace elements in medicine and biology* 37 (2016): 125–133.

8. Heijmans, Bastiaan T., Elmar W. Tobi, Aryeh D. Stein, Hein Putter, Gerard J. Blauw, Ezra S. Susser, P. Eline Slagboom, and L. H. Lumey. "Persistent epigenetic differences associated with prenatal exposure to famine in humans." *Proceedings of the National Academy of Sciences* 105, no. 44 (2008): 17046–17049.

9. Ibid.

10. Vince, Gaia. "Pregnant smokers increases grandkids' asthma risk." *New Scientist*, n.p., 11 Apr. 2005. Web. 12 Oct. 2015. <https://www.newscientist.com/article/dn7252-pregnant-smokers-increases-grandkids-asthma-risk/>.

11. Kanherkar, Riya R., Naina Bhatia-Dey, and Antonei B. Csoka. "Epigenetics across the human lifespan." *Frontiers in cell and developmental biology* 2 (2014): 49.

12. Richardson, Bruce. "DNA methylation and autoimmune disease." *Clinical immunology* 109, no. 1 (2003): 72–79.

13. Reddy, Marpadga A., Erli Zhang, and Rama Natarajan. "Epigenetic mechanisms in diabetic complications and metabolic memory." *Diabetologia* 58, no. 3 (2015): 443–455.

14. Dawson, Mark A., and Tony Kouzarides. "Cancer epigenetics: from mechanism to therapy." *Cell* 150, no. 1 (2012): 12–27.

15. Martínez, J. Alfredo, Fermín I. Milagro, Kate J. Claycombe, and Kevin L. Schalinske. "Epigenetics in adipose tissue, obesity, weight loss, and diabetes." *Advances in nutrition: an international review journal* 5, no. 1 (2014): 71–81.

16. Bayan, Leyla, Peir Hossain Koulivand, and Ali Gorji. "Garlic: a review of potential therapeutic effects." *Avicenna journal of phytomedicine* 4, no. 1 (2014): 1–14.

17. Lenucci, Marcello S., Daniela Cadinu, Marco Taurino, Gabriella Piro, and Giuseppe Dalessandro. "Antioxidant composition in cherry and high-pigment tomato cultivars." *Journal of agricultural and food chemistry* 54, no. 7 (2006): 2606–2613.

18. Davis, Donald R. "Declining fruit and vegetable nutrient composition: what is the evidence?" *HortScience* 44, no. 1 (2009): 15–19.

19. Rickman, Joy C., Diane M. Barrett, and Christine M. Bruhn. "Nutritional comparison of fresh, frozen and canned fruits and vegetables. Part 1. Vitamins C and B and phenolic compounds." *Journal of the science of food and agriculture* 87, no. 6 (2007): 930–944.

Chapter 7

1. Cordain, Loren, S. Boyd Eaton, Anthony Sebastian, Neil Mann, Staffan Lindeberg, Bruce A. Watkins, James H. O'Keefe, and Janette Brand-Miller. "Origins and evolution of the Western diet: health implications for the 21st century." *American journal of clinical nutrition* 81, no. 2 (2005): 341–354.

2. Cordain, Loren, Janette Brand-Miller, S. Boyd Eaton, Neil Mann, Susanne H. A. Holt, and John D. Speth. "Plant-animal subsistence ratios and macronutrient energy estimations in worldwide hunter-gatherer diets." *American journal of clinical nutrition* 71, no. 3 (2000): 682–692.

3. Whips, Heather. "How sugar changed the world." *LiveScience.* 02 June 2008. Web. 11 Dec. 2016. <http://www.livescience.com/4949-sugar-changed-world.html>.

4. Welsh, Jean A., Andrea Sharma, Solveig A. Cunningham, and Miriam B. Vos. "Consumption of added sugars and indicators of cardiovascular disease risk among US adolescents." *Circulation* 123, no. 3 (2011): 249–257.

5. Ervin, R. Bethene, and Cynthia L. Ogden. "Consumption of added sugars among US adults, 2005–2010." *NCHS data brief* 122 (2013): 1-8.

6. Ng, Shu Wen, Meghan M. Slining, and Barry M. Popkin. "Use of caloric and noncaloric sweeteners in US consumer packaged foods, 2005–2009." *Journal of the Academy of Nutrition and Dietetics* 112, no. 11 (2012): 1828–1834.

7. Weiss, Ehud, Wilma Wetterstrom, Dani Nadel, and Ofer Bar-Yosef. "The broad spectrum revisited: evidence from plant remains." *Proceedings of the National Academy of Sciences* 101, no. 26 (2004): 9551–9555.

8. Heshe, G. G., G. D. Haki, A. Z. Woldegiorgis, and H. F. Gemede. "Effect of conventional milling on the nutritional value and antioxidant capacity of wheat types common in Ethiopia and a recovery attempt with bran supplementation in bread." *Food Science & Nutrition* 4 (2016): 534–543.

9. "FAO cereal supply and demand brief." Food and Agriculture Organization of the United Nations, n.p., n.d. Web. 13 Dec. 2016. <http://www.fao.org/worldfoodsituation/csdb/en/>.

10. Riddle, Mark S., Joseph A. Murray, and Chad K. Porter. "The incidence and risk of celiac disease in a healthy US adult population." *American journal of gastroenterology* 107, no. 8 (2012): 1248–1255.

11. Rubio–Tapia, Alberto, Robert A. Kyle, Edward L. Kaplan, Dwight R. Johnson, William Page, Frederick Erdtmann, Tricia L. Brantner, et al. "Increased prevalence and mortality in undiagnosed celiac disease." *Gastroenterology* 137, no. 1 (2009): 88–93.

12. Lionetti, Elena, Stefania Castellaneta, Ruggiero Francavilla, Alfredo Pulvirenti, Elio Tonutti, Sergio Amarri, Maria Barbato, et al. "Introduction of gluten, HLA status, and the risk of celiac disease in children." *New England journal of medicine* 371, no. 14 (2014): 1295–1303.

13. Vriezinga, Sabine L., Renata Auricchio, Enzo Bravi, Gemma Castillejo, Anna Chmielewska, Paula Crespo Escobar, Sanja Kola—ek, et al. "Randomized feeding intervention in infants at high risk for celiac disease." *New England journal of medicine* 371, no. 14 (2014): 1304–1315.

14. Fasano, Alessio. "Zonulin, regulation of tight junctions, and autoimmune diseases." *Annals of the New York Academy of Sciences* 1258, no. 1 (2012): 25–33.

15. Dubey, Rajendra Kumar, Deepesh Kumar Gupta, and Amit Kumar Singh. "Dental implant survival in diabetic patients: review and recommendations." *National journal of maxillofacial surgery* 4, no. 2 (2013): 142.

16. Sun, Sam Z., and Mark W. Empie. "Fructose metabolism in humans—what isotopic tracer studies tell us." *Nutrition & metabolism* 9, no. 1 (2012): 1.

17. Mozaffarian, D., A. Aro, and W. C. Willett. "Health effects of trans-fatty acids: experimental and observational evidence." *European journal of clinical nutrition* 63 (2009): S5–S21.

18. Young, Adam. "The war on margarine." Atlanta, GA. Foundation for Economic Education, June 2002.

19. Jackson, Michael, and Gary List. "Giants of the past: the battle over hydrogenation (1903–1920)", *Inform* 18 (2007): 403–405.

20. Canola   a new oilseed from Canada. *Journal of the American Oil Chemists' Society*, September 1981: 723A–9A.

21. Charlton, K. M., A. H. Corner, K. Davey, J. K. Kramer, S. Mahadevan, and F. D. Sauer. "Cardiac lesions in rats fed rapeseed oils." *Canadian journal of comparative medicine* 39, no. 3 (1975): 261.

22. Wahlqvist, Mark L. "From 'lactose intolerance' to 'lactose nutrition.'" *Asia pac j clin nutr* 24, no. 1 (2015): S1–S8.

23. Curry, Andrew. "Archaeology: the milk revolution." *Nature.com*. Macmillan, 31 July 2013. Web. 12 Dec. 2014. <http://www.nature.com/news/archaeology-the-milk-revolution-1.13471>.

24. Leonardi, M., P. Gerbault, M. G. Thomas, and J. Burger. "The evolution of lactase persistence in Europe. A synthesis of archaeological and genetic evidence." *Int. dairy j.* 22, 88–97 (2012).

25. Holsinger, V. H., K. T. Rajkowski, and J. R. Stabel. "Milk pasteurisation and safety: a brief history and update." *Revue scientifique et technique—office international des epizooties* 16 (1997): 441–466.

26. Jami, Elie, Bryan A. White, and Itzhak Mizrahi. "Potential role of the bovine rumen microbiome in modulating milk composition and feed efficiency." *PLoS One* 9, no. 1 (2014): e85423.

27. Laporte, Marie-France, and Paul Paquin. "Near-infrared analysis of fat, protein, and casein in cow's milk." *Journal of agricultural and food chemistry* 47, no. 7 (1999): 2600–2605.

28. Shackelford, S. D., M. Koohmaraie, and T. L. Wheeler. "Effects of slaughter age on meat tenderness and USDA carcass maturity scores of beef females." *Journal of animal science* 73, no. 11 (1995): 3304–3309.

29. Davies, Julian, and Dorothy Davies. "Origins and evolution of antibiotic resistance." *Microbiology and molecular biology reviews* 74, no. 3 (2010): 417–433.

30. Leheska, J. M., L. D. Thompson, J. C. Howe, E. Hentges, J. Boyce, J. C. Brooks, B. Shriver, L. Hoover, and M. F. Miller. "Effects of conventional and grass-feeding systems on the nutrient composition of beef." *Journal of animal science* 86, no. 12 (2008): 3575–3585.

31. Daley, Cynthia A., Amber Abbott, Patrick S. Doyle, Glenn A. Nader, and Stephanie Larson. "A review of fatty acid profiles and antioxidant content in grass-fed and grain-fed beef." *Nutrition journal* 9, no. 1 (2010): 1.

32. Cordain, Loren, S. Boyd Eaton, Anthony Sebastian, Neil Mann, Staffan Lindeberg, Bruce A. Watkins, James H. O'Keefe, and Janette Brand-Miller. "Origins and evolution of the Western diet: health implications for the 21st century." *American journal of clinical nutrition* 81, no. 2 (2005): 341–354.

33. Selhub, Eva M., Alan C. Logan, and Alison C. Bested. "Fermented foods, microbiota, and mental health: ancient practice meets nutritional psychiatry." *Journal of physiological anthropology* 33, no. 1 (2014): 1.

Chapter 8

1. Ng, Marie, Tom Fleming, Margaret Robinson, Blake Thomson, Nicholas Graetz, Christopher Margono, Erin C. Mullany, et al. "Global, regional, and national prevalence of overweight and obesity in children and adults during 1980–2013: a systematic analysis for the Global Burden of Disease Study 2013." *Lancet* 384, no. 9945 (2014): 766–781.

2. Keys, Ancel, Alessandro Mienotti, Mariti J. Karvonen, Christ Aravanis, Henry Blackburn, Ratko Buzina, B. S. Djordjevic, et al. "The diet and 15-year death rate in the seven countries study." *American journal of epidemiology* 124, no. 6 (1986): 903–915.

3. Stamler, J. "Diet–heart: a problematic revisit." *American journal of clinical nutrition* 91, no. 3 (2010): 497–499.

4. Hite, Adele H., Richard David Feinman, Gabriel E. Guzman, Morton Satin, Pamela A. Schoenfeld, and Richard J. Wood. "In the face of contradictory evidence: report of the Dietary Guidelines for Americans Committee." *Nutrition* 26, no. 10 (2010): 915–924.

5. Ravnskov, Uffe. "The fallacies of the lipid hypothesis." *Scandinavian cardiovascular journal* 42, no. 4 (2008): 236–239.

6. Ford, Earl S., Umed A. Ajani, Janet B. Croft, Julia A. Critchley, Darwin R. Labarthe, Thomas E. Kottke, Wayne H. Giles, and Simon Capewell. "Explaining the decrease in US deaths from coronary disease, 1980–2000." *New England journal of medicine* 356, no. 23 (2007): 2388–2398.

7. Finkelstein, Eric A., Olga A. Khavjou, Hope Thompson, Justin G. Trogdon, Liping Pan, Bettylou Sherry, and William Dietz. "Obesity and severe obesity forecasts through 2030." *American journal of preventive medicine* 42, no. 6 (2012): 563–570.

8. Lam, David W., and Derek LeRoith. "The worldwide diabetes epidemic." *Current opinion in endocrinology, diabetes and obesity* 19, no. 2 (2012): 93–96.

9. Siri-Tarino, Patty W., Qi Sun, Frank B. Hu, and Ronald M. Krauss. "Meta-analysis of prospective cohort studies evaluating the association of saturated fat with cardiovascular disease." *American journal of clinical nutrition 91* (2010): 535–46.

10. Chowdhury, Rajiv, Samantha Warnakula, Setor Kunutsor, Francesca Crowe, Heather A. Ward, Laura Johnson, Oscar H. Franco, et al. "Association of dietary, circulating, and supplement fatty acids with coronary risk: a systematic review and meta-analysis." *Annals of internal medicine* 160, no. 6 (2014): 398–406.

11. Sachdeva, Amit, Christopher P. Cannon, Prakash C. Deedwania, Kenneth A. LaBresh, Sidney C. Smith, David Dai, Adrian Hernandez, and Gregg C. Fonarow. "Lipid levels in patients hospitalized with coronary artery disease: an analysis of 136,905 hospitalizations in Get with the Guidelines." *American heart journal* 157, no. 1 (2009): 111–117.

12. Dreon, Darlene M., Harriett A. Fernstrom, Hannia Campos, Patricia Blanche, Paul T. Williams, and Ronald M. Krauss. "Change in dietary saturated fat intake is correlated with change in mass of large low-density-lipoprotein particles in men." *American journal of clinical nutrition* 67, no. 5 (1998): 828–836.

13. Siri-Tarino, Patty W., Qi Sun, Frank B. Hu, and Ronald M. Krauss. "Saturated fat, carbohydrate, and cardiovascular disease." *American journal of clinical nutrition* 91, no. 3 (2010): 502–509.

14. Berger, Samantha, Gowri Raman, Rohini Vishwanathan, Paul F. Jacques, and Elizabeth J. Johnson. "Dietary cholesterol and cardiovascular disease: a systematic review and meta-analysis." *American journal of clinical nutrition* 102 (2015): 276–94.

15. National Institutes of Health. "Lowering blood cholesterol to prevent heart disease." U.S. Department of Health and Human Services, 10 Dec. 1984. Web. 13 Aug. 2015. <https://consensus.nih.gov/1984/1984cholesterol047html.htm>.

16. For the term "Snackwell's phenomenon," see Tamar Haspel, "Stealth shopping: insider tips for finding and buying the healthiest groceries," *Prevention*, February 2005, 57, 208. The actual product name is SnackWell's.

17. Hazan, Marcella. *The Essentials of Classic Italian Cooking.* London: Boxtree, 2011.

18. Bang, H. O., J. Dyerberg, and Hugh Macdonald Sinclair. "The composition of the Eskimo food in north western Greenland." *American journal of clinical nutrition* 33, no. 12 (1980): 2657–2661.

19. Kris-Etherton, Penny M., William S. Harris, and Lawrence J. Appel. "Fish consumption, fish oil, omega-3 fatty acids, and cardiovascular disease." *Circulation* 106, no. 21 (2002): 2747–2757.

20. Mohebi-Nejad, Azin, and Behnood Bikdeli. "Omega-3 supplements and cardiovascular diseases." *Tanaffos* 13, no. 1 (2014): 6.

21. Simopoulos, Artemis P. "The importance of the ratio of omega-6/omega-3 essential fatty acids." *Biomedicine & pharmacotherapy* 56, no. 8 (2002): 365–379.

22. "What Is Cholesterol?" *National Heart Lung and Blood Institute*, U.S. Department of Health and Human Services, 12 Nov. 2013, www.nhlbi.nih.gov/health/health-topics/topics/hbc/. Accessed 10 June 2016.

23. Lecerf, Jean-Michel, and Michel De Lorgeril. "Dietary cholesterol: from physiology to cardiovascular risk." *British journal of nutrition* 106, no. 1 (2011): 6–14.

24. Tulenko, Thomas N., and Anne E. Sumner. "The physiology of lipoproteins." *Journal of nuclear cardiology* 9, no. 6 (2002): 638–649.

25. Griffin, John D., and Alice H. Lichtenstein. "Dietary cholesterol and plasma lipoprotein profiles: randomized controlled trials." *Current nutrition reports* 2, no. 4 (2013): 274–282.

26. Preshaw, P. M., A. L. Alba, D. Herrera, S. Jepsen, A. Konstantinidis, K. Makrilakis, and R. Taylor. "Periodontitis and diabetes: a two-way relationship." *Diabetologia* 55, no. 1 (2012): 21–31.

27. Centers for Disease Control and Prevention. "National diabetes statistics report: estimates of diabetes and its burden in the United States, 2014." Atlanta, GA: US Department of Health and Human Services 2014.

28. Taylor, Roy. "Insulin resistance and type 2 diabetes." *Diabetes* 61, no. 4 (2012): 778–779.

29. Basaranoglu, Metin, Gokcen Basaranoglu, and Elisabetta Bugianesi. "Carbohydrate intake and nonalcoholic fatty liver disease: fructose as a weapon of mass destruction." *Hepatobiliary Surgery and Nutrition.* 4, no. 2 (2015): 109–116.

30. Calvo, Carlos, Corinne Talussot, Gabriel Ponsin, and Francois Berthézène. "Non enzymatic glycation of apolipoprotein AI. Effects on its self-association and lipid binding properties." *Biochemical and biophysical research communications* 153, no. 3 (1988): 1060–1067.

31. Bucala, Richard, Zenji Makita, Gloria Vega, Scott Grundy, Theodor Koschinsky, Anthony Cerami, and Helen Vlassara. "Modification of low density lipoprotein by advanced glycation end products contributes to the dyslipidemia of diabetes and renal insufficiency." *Proceedings of the National Academy of Sciences* 91, no. 20 (1994): 9441–9445.

32. Yang, Quanhe, Zefeng Zhang, Edward W. Gregg, W. Dana Flanders, Robert Merritt, and Frank B. Hu. "Added sugar intake and cardiovascular diseases mortality among US adults." *JAMA internal medicine* 174, no. 4 (2014): 516–524.

33. Basciano, Heather, Lisa Federico, and Khosrow Adeli. "Fructose, insulin resistance, and metabolic dyslipidemia." *Nutrition & metabolism* 2, no. 1 (2005): 5.

34. Ahmed, Monjur. "Non-alcoholic fatty liver disease in 2015." *World journal of hepatology* 7, no. 11 (2015): 1450–1459.

35. Lustig, Robert H., Kathleen Mulligan, Susan M. Noworolski, Viva W. Tai, Michael J. Wen, Ayca Erkin-Cakmak, Alejandro Gugliucci, and Jean-Marc Schwarz. "Isocaloric fructose restriction and metabolic improvement in children with obesity and metabolic syndrome." *Obesity* 24, no. 2 (2016): 453–460.

Chapter 9

1. Sonnenburg, Justin L., and Fredrik Bäckhed. "Diet–microbiota interactions as moderators of human metabolism." *Nature* 535, 56–64 (2016).

2. Porges, Stephen W., and Senta A. Furman. "The early development of the autonomic nervous system provides a neural platform for social behaviour: a polyvagal perspective." *Infant and child development* 20, no. 1 (2011): 106–118.

3. Peres, Karen Glazer, Andreia Morales Cascaes, Marco Aurelio Peres, Flavio Fernando Demarco, Iná Silva Santos, Alicia Matijasevich, and Aluisio J. D. Barros. "Exclusive breastfeeding and risk of dental malocclusion." *Pediatrics* 136, no. 1 (2015): e60–e67.

4. Mulligan, Megan L., Shaili K. Felton, Amy E. Riek, and Carlos Bernal-Mizrachi. "Implications of vitamin D deficiency in pregnancy and lactation." *American journal of obstetrics and gynecology* 202, no. 5 (2010): 429–e1.

5. Jost, Ted, Christophe Lacroix, Christian P. Braegger, Florence Rochat, and Christophe Chassard. "Vertical mother–neonate transfer of maternal gut bacteria via breastfeeding." *Environmental microbiology* 16, no. 9 (2014): 2891–2904.

6. Verduci, Elvira, Giuseppe Banderali, Salvatore Barberi, Giovanni Radaelli, Alessandra Lops, Federica Betti, Enrica Riva, and Marcello Giovannini. "Epigenetic effects of human breast milk." *Nutrients* 6, no. 4 (2014): 1711–1724.

7. Chivasa, Stephen, Bongani K. Ndimba, William J. Simon, Keith Lindsey, and Antoni R. Slabas. "Extracellular ATP functions as an endogenous external metabolite regulating plant cell viability." *Plant cell* 17, no. 11 (2005): 3019–3034.

8. Zittermann, Armin. "Magnesium deficit—overlooked cause of low vitamin D status?" *BMC medicine* 11, no. 1 (2013): 1.

9. Jackson, Kelly A., Ruth A. Valentine, Lisa J. Coneyworth, John C. Mathers, and Dianne Ford. "Mechanisms of mammalian zinc-regulated gene expression." *Biochemical Society transactions* 36, no. 6 (2008): 1262–1266.

10. Christian, Parul, and K. P. West. "Interactions between zinc and vitamin A: an update." *American journal of clinical nutrition* 68, no. 2 (1998): 435S–441S.

11. Kasai, Kikuo, Masami Kobayashi, and Shin-Ichi Shimoda. "Stimulatory effect of glycine on human growth hormone secretion." *Metabolism* 27, no. 2 (1978): 201–208.

Chapter 10

1. Scrimshaw, Nevin S., and Edwina B. Murray. "The acceptability of milk and milk products in populations with a high prevalence of lactose intolerance." *American journal of clinical nutrition* 48, no. 4 (1988): 1142–1159.

INDEX

Note: Page numbers in *italics* indicate recipes.

A

Acid reflux, 54
Activator X
    dubbing of, 25
    hunt for, 68–72
    vitamin K2 as, 70–71, 76, 77
Adenosine triphosphate (ATP), 183
ADHD, 16, 33, 54–56, 102
Aiello, Leslie C., 35
Alcohol, 99, 147, 189
Alcoholism, 114, 166
Allergies, 102, 137, 216
Allicin, 122
Alternate nostril breathing exercise, 250
Alveolar nerve, 40
Alzheimer's disease, 52, 66, 102
American Association of Oral and Maxillofacial Surgeons, 32
American Heart Journal, 153
Ancestral eating, 145–146
Ancestral health, 279
Animal fats, 28, 186, 219
Animalcules, 83
Antibiotics, 84, 99, 124, 144, 179
Anxiety, 52, 54
Apple cider vinegar, 229
Appositional growth, 45
Asian-Style Seafood Soup with Zucchini and Carrot Noodles, *267*
Autism, 16
Autoimmune disease, 100–101, 120, 178
Avocados
    about: oil, 220
    Avocado Cauliflower
    Tabbouleh, *260–261*
    Avocado Egg Boats, *254*
    Avocado Mousse, *248*
    Avocado Soup, *265*
    Zesty Pepper Chicken Wings with Sweet Potato Chips and Guacamole, *245*

B

Bacteria. *See also* Microbes; Microbiome
    bacterial gene sequencing, 15
    fiber for healthy mouth and gut, 99
    health dictated by, 92–95
    managing minerals in teeth, 88–90
    metabolizing, 176
    mouth needing, 87–90
    probiotic, 95–96, 176, 192
    role in tooth decay, 82
Baked Vegetables, *202*
Balance step of Dental Diet Program, 191–192
Beef Broth, *210–211*
Beef Liver Steak, *235–236*
Bikini bodies, 154
Bile, 182
Biodiversity, 86–87
Biofilm, 88, 89
Bleeding gums, 97–102, 164
Bloating, 52, 54, 137, 216
Blood cells, 64, 65
Blubber, 30, 160
Blueberry Chia Pudding, *258*
The Blue Zones (Buettner), 157
Bone density, 67, 182
Bone marrow, 64, 65
Braces, 12

ACKNOWLEDGMENTS

When I embarked on the journey of writing this book, I had no idea just how challenging and life-changing an experience it would be. As a health care professional, we are tragically ill-equipped with the knowledge or skills to enter the publishing world. Dentistry, in particular, is not an area well known for its literary prowess. So to the following people, I would like to thank you wholeheartedly.

Posthumously I send my gratitude and appreciation to Weston A. Price. The powerful and inspiring conviction of his work was capable of waking me from a robot-like view of dental health. It's an honor to write his name, and I sincerely hope that this book helps to get his work the recognition it so desperately deserves.

To the people at the Price-Pottenger and Weston A. Price Foundation, I thank you for your kindness and good work in allowing Price's work to live on and for your assistance in materials for this book.

Along the way, I have spoken to countless people working on truly innovative aspects of their field. Unfortunately, many of these conversations could not be in the final version, which was a difficult pill to swallow each time. I wish to thank every person along the way who has contributed through the inspiration of their ideas and work.

To Cassie Hanjian, my literary agent, for her laser-like vision and skills to see that a dental health book was both possible and needed. Your work ethic and "hustle" was the breath of life that *The Dental Diet* needed. I am so happy to have met and gone through this process with you.

To the Hay House office in New York, Patty Gift and the team. Firstly for being such an open-minded and caring group of people. Secondly for believing an Australian dentist that there was indeed a book-worthy concept here. Lisa Cheng, my editor who pored over the work with such oversight and refinement, every little thought has been like gold.

As this book sits in front of me, I can't escape the picture of thousands of pages of hieroglyphic-like scientific studies and essays painstakingly translated into what it is today. My most sincere thanks to Colby Brin for his invaluable assistance and generous support in the preparation of this manuscript. Your guidance, wisdom, and insight helped to make this book a reality.

To the team at Kingsgrove Dental, for your patience and support during this unconventional process. Without your understanding and flexibility, this would never have been possible.

And finally to my family, for your love and support without which I simply would not be here today.

ABOUT THE AUTHOR

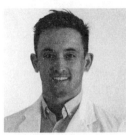 **Dr. Steven Lin** is a board-accredited dentist, speaker, and author. Frustrated by the dental profession's limited approach to applying treatments without addressing the cause of disease, Dr. Lin merged anthropological, physiological, and nutritional science with oral health to integrate effective prevention strategies into his dental practice. A passionate health educator, Dr. Lin engages in a wide variety of community and institutional programs to increase awareness of preventative lifestyles. He is the dental expert for *I Quit Sugar*, the online platform of best-selling author Sarah Wilson. Dr. Lin's speaking and training programs have been delivered all over the world, and you can visit him online at www.drstevenlin.com and on social media @drstevenlin.

We hope you enjoyed this Hay House book. If you'd like to
receive our online catalog featuring additional information
on Hay House books and products, or if you'd like to find
out more about the Hay Foundation, please contact:

Hay House, Inc., P.O. Box 5100,
Carlsbad, CA 92018-5100
(760) 431-7695 or (800) 654-5126
(760) 431-6948 (fax) or (800) 650-5115 (fax)
www.hayhouse.com® • www.hayfoundation.org

◆ ◆ ◆

Published and distributed in Australia by: Hay House Australia Pty. Ltd.,
18/36 Ralph St., Alexandria NSW 2015 • *Phone:* 612-9669-4299
Fax: 612-9669-4144 • www.hayhouse.com.au

Published and distributed in the United Kingdom by: Hay House UK, Ltd.,
Astley House, 33 Notting Hill Gate, London W11 3JQ • *Phone:* 44-20-3675-2450
Fax: 44-20-3675-2451 • www.hayhouse.co.uk

Published in India by: Hay House Publishers India, Muskaan Complex,
Plot No. 3, B-2, Vasant Kunj, New Delhi 110 070 • *Phone:* 91-11-4176-1620
Fax: 91-11-4176-1630 • www.hayhouse.co.in

Distributed in Canada by: Raincoast Books, 2440 Viking Way, Richmond, B.C.
V6V 1N2 • *Phone:* 1-800-663-5714 • *Fax:* 1-800-565-3770 • www.raincoast.com

◆ ◆ ◆

Access New Knowledge.
Anytime. Anywhere.

Learn and evolve at your own pace with the world's leading experts.

www.hayhouseU.com

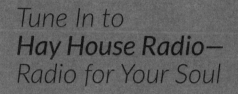